Dr. Chris's A, B, C's of Health

When your body screams, listen to it!

Chris Elisabeth Gilbert, M.D., Ph.D.

iUniverse, Inc.
New York Bloomington

Dr. Chris's A, B, C's of Health
When your body screams, listen to it!

iUniverse books may be ordered through booksellers or by contacting:

iUniverse
1663 Liberty Drive
Bloomington, IN 47403
www.iuniverse.com
1-800-Authors (1-800-288-4677)

Because of the dynamic nature of the Internet, any Web addresses or links contained in this book may have changed since publication and may no longer be valid. The views expressed in this work are solely those of the author and do not necessarily reflect the views of the publisher, and the publisher hereby disclaims any responsibility for them.

ISBN: 978-1-4502-4816-7 (sc)
ISBN: 978-1-4502-4817-4 (ebook)

Printed in the United States of America

iUniverse rev. date: 9/10/2010

A concise guide on how to stay healthy and happy for the rest of your life.

Acknowledgments

To my father Jacques, who was a wonderful physician and taught me how to listen to each patient and find the best treatment for every single one of them regardless of the time it took.

To my mother Jacqueline, who taught me how to respect and try to understand every single individual regardless of his or her age, gender, nationality, race, religion and past.

To my husband Steve, the love of my life, whose strength and sense of humor brightened each of my days for 12 wonderful years and who made me a better human being.

To all my friends and family members whose support has been strong throughout the years.

Thanks to all the people who participated in the editing, drawings and photography for this book.

Editing: Above all, my husband Steve Chmura. Also Richard Forest and Evelyn Goodwin.

Drawings: My mother Jacqueline Gilbert.

Photography: Pierre Colin.

In loving memory of the two most wonderful men of my life, my father Jacques and my husband Steve.

In medicine there is no guarantee. The information provided in this book is offered for educational purposes only.

The information in this book does not create a physician-patient relationship between you and Dr. Gilbert.

Dr. Gilbert does not guarantee the accuracy or completeness of any information available in this book.

You must check with your personal physician to assess whether suggestions herein are appropriate for you since results will vary among individuals and there could be substantial risks involved.

Table of Contents

Introduction

"It is easy to get a thousand prescriptions but hard to get one single remedy."

Chinese proverb

Most physicians and insurance companies think that medicine is simple. They think that 15 minutes per patient are enough to ask questions, examine the patient, make a diagnosis and prescribe appropriate medications. Well, after 30 years of practicing medicine, my conclusion is that medicine is not that simple. Fifteen minutes with each patient are not enough. Prescribing a painkiller, an antidepressant, a sleeping pill or a stomach medication is just addressing the tip of the iceberg.

What is lying deep inside? Why are you fatigued? Why are you in pain? Why are you depressed? Why can't you sleep at night? Why are you sick all the time? Those are the questions that need to be answered.

Some of us have a genetic defect which is difficult to correct but most of us don't. Most people are in chronic pain or are sick all the time because they have unhealthy habits.

Chances are you are eating the wrong foods, drinking the wrong beverages and not exercising enough. Chances are you hate your job, you are married to the wrong person and you live in a place you don't like.

There is a very strong mind-body interaction and if your mind is unhappy, you will get sick. If you eat the wrong food and exercise the wrong way, your body will get sick. There could be irreversible damage and since longevity is at an all time high, you could be in pain for many years. It is never too late to start over. I did it myself and I'll show you how to do it in this book. The key is to treat your body as a whole. The science is called Holistic Medicine.

I want you to have a healthy body and mind. Here is how to do it.

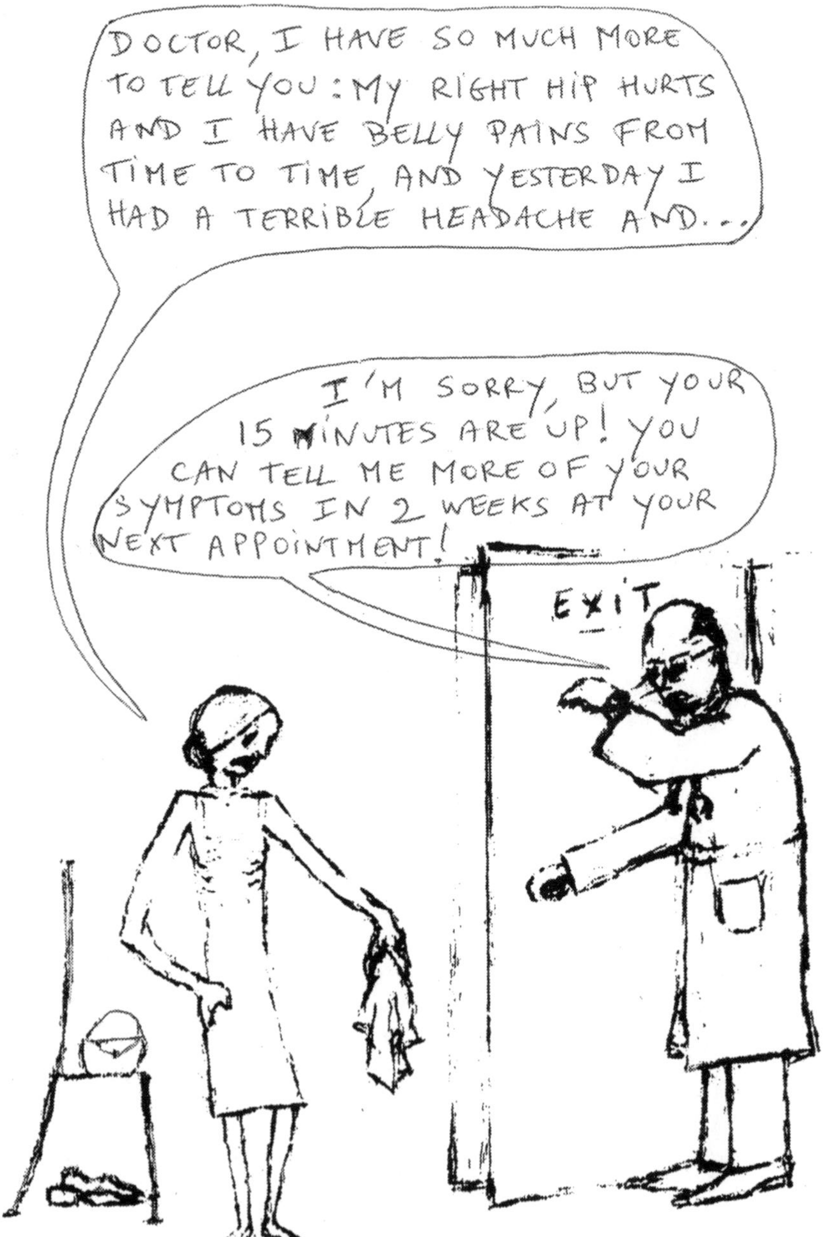
DOCTOR, I HAVE SO MUCH MORE TO TELL YOU: MY RIGHT HIP HURTS AND I HAVE BELLY PAINS FROM TIME TO TIME, AND YESTERDAY I HAD A TERRIBLE HEADACHE AND...
I'M SORRY, BUT YOUR 15 MINUTES ARE UP! YOU CAN TELL ME MORE OF YOUR SYMPTOMS IN 2 WEEKS AT YOUR NEXT APPOINTMENT!
EXIT

Chapter 1
Living a healthy life is like surfing the waves while spinning all our plates at a perfectly balanced speed.

"When the student is ready, the master appears"

Buddhist proverb

Have you ever been to a circus? Have you ever seen an entertainer spinning plates? Well, my deep belief is that living a healthy life is like surfing the waves while spinning all our main plates at a perfectly balanced speed. This is very difficult to do. But first let me explain in more detail what that means.

Our body is born pretty close to perfect. Each cell has a purpose and is interconnected with all the others. Our body is a work of art. We need to take good care of it. It is very easy to harm it. In order to keep it functioning the right way, we need to be like an acrobat spinning plates. We need to spin each plate every day at the right balanced speed for us. The plates that need to be spun every day are:

- Foods: Eat the right foods at the right time
- Beverages: Drink the right beverages
- Breathe good quality air

- Sleep regular hours
- Exercise the right way every day
- Spend quality time by ourselves
- Spend pleasant time with family and friends
- Have a goal in life and work on achieving it

While we are doing this, life changes, it makes waves so we need to learn how to surf each wave the best way possible while continuing to spin all our plates.

Every day, we are interacting with people who are also surfing their own waves and trying to spin their own plates. A lot of people are not good at doing this and their plates fall all over around us before they fall themselves.

We then need to learn how to surf our waves while spinning our plates in a balanced way, being surrounded by plates and people falling all around us. That is what I call learning life!

Chapter 2
First Do No Harm!

"Don't dig your grave with your own knife and fork."

English proverb

First Do No Harm or in Latin Primum Non Nocere! Although this is not in the Hippocratic Oath, it is one of the principal precepts all medical students are taught in medical school. It should be the same first rule for each one of us to take care of our own body. Our body is so delicate! It is so easy to damage it. First do not harm it!

Your body needs a balanced diet. Do not harm it by eating the wrong foods like too many high fat fast-food meals. Do not eat too many cookies, cakes, sweets and ice cream otherwise you'll get cavities in your teeth, you'll clog up your arteries, you might get diabetes and be prone to infections.

Do not harm it by drinking the wrong beverages otherwise you'll increase your chances of having heart disease (too many regular sweet soft drinks) or liver disease (too much alcohol).

Do not harm it by smoking otherwise you might get lung cancer or heart disease. "Just a pack a day" represents 200 inhalations of poison per day and more than 70,000 inhalations of poison a year.

The poison gases are carbon monoxide, ammonia, formaldehyde and cyanide. Carbon monoxide is what kills people when they leave the car engine running in the garage. Ammonia is the same chemical found in urine and household cleaners. Formaldehyde is used to preserve body parts. Cyanide is used to execute those convicted of capital offenses. You might as well be breathing bus exhaust gases! A lot of cigarette smokers also get COPD which stands for chronic obstructive pulmonary disease. Their lungs cannot function well any more and they get chronically short of breath. As for chewing tobacco or smoking the pipe, it puts people at risk of cancer of the mouth or throat.

Do not harm your body by taking street drugs otherwise you might damage your brain. Illegal drugs are illegal for a reason. Some drugs like cocaine and methamphetamine can give heart attacks and sudden death. MDMA (3,4-ethylenedioxymethamphetamine), or ecstasy is been responsible for memory deficits, high fevers, liver failure, coronary spasms and death. Morphine can give respiratory arrest and also sudden death.

Do not harm it by taking too many over-the-counter drugs: Acetaminophen (contained in Tylenol) everyday could damage your liver; Ibuprofen everyday could give you stomach ulcers and make you bleed to death. As for prescription drugs, they require a prescription for a reason. They can be very dangerous if used for the wrong problems and used at a higher dosage. Vicodin, Darvocet, Percocet, Norco, Tylenol # 3 for example are addictive and could interact with other medications. If used too much and too frequently, they could cause liver failure.

Do not harm your body by staying at your computer for 8 or 10 hours in a row without moving. It could clog your arteries. On the other hand, do not overstress your joints, it could damage them.

Do not harm your body by sleeping too little and being under too much stress otherwise you might damage your hormonal production and the connections between your brain cells.

Do not harm your body by laying hours in the sun between 10.00am to 3:00pm without adequate sunscreen protection. It could give you skin cancer. On the other hand, do not harm it by never being outside otherwise your body won't produce enough Vitamin D. 15 minutes per day in the sun is the time needed for you body to produce the right amount of this essential hormone.

Do not harm your body by hanging out with the wrong friends, by marrying the wrong partner or starting the wrong job. You'll damage your neurons' electrical circuits.

You have much more power over your life than you think you have. You are just not aware of it and not using it.

Chris Elisabeth Gilbert, M.D., Ph.D.

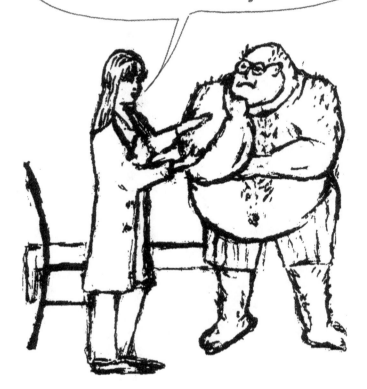

Chapter 3
When your body screams, listen to it!

"In a time of drastic change, it is the learners *who inherit the future. The* learned *find themselves equipped to live in a world that no longer exists."*

Eric Hoffer

"It is astonishing what happens when we approach everything with kindness! When we approach a pain with kindness, it can have a voice, talk and say stunning things! The key is to be completely open to anything and everything, welcoming the unknown and discovering with awe the amazing world of the subconscious."

Chris Gilbert, MD, PhD

Your body actually talks to you all the time. Did you notice? Can you spend a few minutes a day listening to your body? What if those aches and pains you are having were actually your body talking to you? What if your body wanted to communicate with you, tell you that you are doing something wrong? What if your body knew how to fix itself and wanted you to listen to it? How would your body do this? How could it catch your attention? Perhaps by giving you pain!... And if you don't listen to it, by giving you more and more pain until you are forced to listen to it... Could that be possible? My answer is yes!

What about dreams? Could your body tell you what to do and not to do through recurrent dreams? My answer is sometimes!

The powerful technique of being in the present moment, aware of sensations, emotions and behaviors is called Gestalt Therapy. The German term Gestalt refers to something that has been "put together." Gestalt Therapy was developed by Fritz Perls in the 1940's. It allows people to access some of the unconscious or repressed part of themselves. Below are some examples.

S. case:

A few months ago, S. came to see me. She was desperately in need of a new treatment. She was 61 years old and had been having neck pain and bilateral shoulder pain for over 5 years. The pain was getting worse every year. Nobody had managed to fix her. She had had X-Rays and CT scans which were all normal. She had tried every type of pill and physical therapy treatment. Nothing had worked! I decided to make her neck and shoulders talk and we created a dialogue between S. and her shoulders.

First I asked her to relax, take a few deep breaths and then make her shoulders talk. I placed a stool in front of her seat to represent her shoulders and I asked her to sit on that stool and talk for her shoulders. Here is what happened:

Shoulders: "We are hurting so much! S. is putting so much pressure on us to do a perfect job at work, then do a perfect job at home, take care of S.'s mother, take care of her husband, children and grandchildren; this is too much for us! We have to work so much! We never have a relaxing moment!"

Then, I asked S. to change seats and switch back to her chair to answer her shoulders:

S: "Really! I am sorry I wasn't aware of this! Anyhow, I do have to take care of everybody. I have no choice." I ask S. to ask her shoulders how to improve them: "what can I do to make you feel better, shoulders?"

I asked her to switch seats again and after a couple of deep breaths:

Shoulders: "We need to have some time off when we have no pressure on us. We need to get in a hot bath and rest. We need you to listen to some relaxing music or do some relaxing reading."

I asked her to switch seats again to answer her shoulders:

"I can definitely do this from time to time. That would actually make me feel better too. What else do you need from me, shoulders?"

Shoulders: "We need you to take care of us, to take care of yourself and slow down! We need you to have a better diet! You eat too much junk food! We are tired and need to rest!"

S. was amazed at how much her shoulders could talk. She decided she would spend at least 30 minutes a day laying down, reading or listening to music, that she would spend less time taking care of her mother, children and grandchildren and more time taking care of herself.

One month later when I saw her, her shoulders and neck were 75% improved.

M. Case:

M. was a 34 year old lady who came to see me because she had been feeling as if she had a lump in her throat for the past 6 months. It all started when she got a new boss at work who was very controlling. The feeling of lump in her throat was getting worse every day. She had seen several ear, nose and throat specialists who weren't able to find anything wrong with her. In desperation, she came to see me.

First again, I made her relax, take deep breaths, then I put a stool in front of her and asked her to seat on that stool to make her throat talk.

Throat: "I feel there is a lump in me, something big that is preventing me from eating, drinking, talking and enjoying life."

I asked her throat to describe her feelings a bit more: "I feel like there is so much pressure under this big mass. This mass is preventing the pressure to release. Pressure is building up but cannot come out. I am so miserable!"

I asked her what the pressure would say if it could talk: "It would say that I hate my new boss. There are so many things I would want to tell him but I can't. I have to keep it all inside."

I asked her throat what it would say if it could:

Throat: "I would say to my boss that he is too controlling and too hard on me. He never compliments me on my work. As soon as I finish a project, there is never any thank you or acknowledgement but there are immediately 2 or 3 more big projects that need to be done within 24 hours. I only have 10 minutes for lunch. I cannot take the pressure. It is way too much. I feel squeezed like a lemon but I cannot say anything because I am afraid of losing my job!"

As M's throat was talking, M started to comment that her throat was starting to relax and that the lump she had been feeling for the last 6 months was starting to go away.

I asked M's throat what would be the solution:

Throat: "M. should ask to be transferred to another department in the same company and she should go for a walk every morning before going to work".

I asked M. if she could do what her throat was suggesting. She said she would try.

One month later, when I saw her, she was waiting to be transferred to another department and she had started walking 15 minutes every morning before going to work. She was feeling much better and the feeling of lump in her throat was almost gone.

B. case:

B. was a 27 year old beautiful and rather big lady who came to me because she was having the same horrifying dream over and over again. She couldn't figure out why and was very apprehensive about going to sleep. One of her doctors had started her on anti-anxiety pills but the dream would still occasionally recur. Her dream was always about a house. It was a big empty house. She was inside and couldn't get out because all the doors were locked from outside. Suddenly a fire started inside one of the rooms. The house was burning down and she was stuck inside. Each time, she would wake up screaming as the flames were getting to her.

I told her there probably was a purpose for the dream to recur. Her body needed to tell her something very important. We started exploring her dream. First I asked her to be the house and describe herself as the house.

House: "I am big, beautiful, made with solid wood. I am sitting on a very large property which is beautiful too. I have a lot of rooms but they are all empty. It seems that nobody lives there. As much as my outside is beautiful, my inside is ugly. The paint of my walls is chipping away but I am still functional with water and electricity."

I asked her to talk about the doors locked:

House: "my doors are all beautiful and strong but they are locked from outside. Nobody can get in and nobody can get out."

I asked B. if the way the house was talking could apply to her life.

B. suddenly burst into tears: "Oh yes, this is me! I am a big woman and I think I was quite beautiful in the past. I do look good from the outside but deep inside, I feel completely empty. I think it comes from my mother who was very dominating and never allowed me to be who I wanted to be and do the things I wanted to do. Even though she passed away 3 years ago, I am still the same as when she was alive."

I asked B. to do another experiment and talk as if she was the fire in her dream:

Fire: "I have red flames. I am strong, violent and fierce. I am so angry! I want to destroy everything on my way! I want to burn all the past so that something new can come from the ashes! I have been repressed a long time but now I am bursting out and I am going to destroy the house."

I asked the fire if it was bad or just cleansing:

Fire: "I am not bad. As a matter of fact, I am quite good! There are a lot of old things that need to be burned and destroyed so that something new and beautiful can be built. I am cleansing."

I explained to B. that the fire was another part of her. It was probably the part that had been repressed for so long and wanted to come out and live. B. was in awe! She had just discovered that 2 very powerful parts of herself were talking in her dream. It wasn't a bad dream. It was a very good dream that had a lot of meaning. She did feel empty inside. It was time to put aside what her mother had taught her. After all she was an adult now. Her mother had been gone for several years. It was time for her to discover who she really was, what she was created on earth for and what her passion was. It was time to get to know her fire inside and not be afraid of it any more. B. was so excited! It was the beginning of a new life for her.

One month later when I saw her again, she was completely off anti-anxiety pills. Her new life had begun. She had decided to learn interior design which is something she always wanted to do but her mother would have been against it. She was a changed woman!

Your turn:

Do you have any recurrent dreams or nightmares? What do they mean?

What symptoms are you feeling that cannot go away or that come back all the time despite all the possible treatments?

What if that part of your body could talk, what would it say?

Chapter 4
Foods

Eat the right foods for your body at the right time of the day.

"To lengthen your life, shorten your meals."

Proverb

67% of adults in the United States are overweight (Body Mass Index - BMI over 25).

33% of adults in the United States are obese (BMI over 30).

To calculate your Body Mass Index, multiply 703 by your weight in lbs and divide this number by your height in inches times 2:

BMI = 703 x Wt (lbs) divide by Ht (inches) x Ht (inches).

Ideally, your BMI should be between 18.5 and 24.9. If your BMI is over 25.0, you are overweight. If it is under 18.5, you are underweight.

Between 1980 and 2000, the number of overweight adolescents tripled and the number of overweight children doubled. As for infants, one third of those born today will develop diabetes. Those numbers are staggering!

The explanation: a lot of high-calorie-cheap-food readily available!

One example: a fast food chain will offer for $3.25 a too-good-to-pass-deal: a burger with 37 grams of fat and 630 calories, 2 tacos with 21 grams of fat and 369 calories, a large portion of fries with 25 grams of fat and 641 calories and a large coke with 499 calories. This makes a total of 83 grams of fat and 2,139 calories which is more than you need for the whole day... and that is only for one meal!

Your body secretes 2 newly discovered hormones: one is called Leptin which is secreted by your fat cells telling your brain to stop eating; the other one is called Ghrelin which is secreted by your stomach telling your brain to eat more. As you get fatter, your body is secreting more and more Leptin which should tell your brain to eat less and less but guess what, all those high-calorie-fast-food diets are making your body resistant to Leptin. It doesn't recognize the signal to stop eating any more. So your body will get fatter and fatter, your fat cells will secrete more and more Leptin, hoping that your brain will get the message. But your brain doesn't get the message so your body gets even fatter to secrete even more Leptin, hoping your brain will finally get it. Your body is screaming that you need to stop eating the wrong foods but your brain still doesn't understand. The food you are eating makes your body completely insensitive to Leptin. That's the problem! How do you fix it?

Well, forget about fast foods, your body needs a balanced diet! Your body needs you to cook! If you don't have time to cook, cook anyways! Cook a large quantity of healthy food once a week, cook enough for the whole week, package everything in small one day's worth containers and freeze them.

Why aren't French people more overweight? Because eating out in France is very expensive so they seldom eat out. Most people cook at home using a lot of healthy ingredients, walking to the stores to get those ingredients and spending time and energy standing up to cook!

Your body needs a balanced diet!

<u>A perfect plate for a meal s</u>hould contain:

One fourth of the plate: whole grains

Half of the plate: fruits and vegetables (include a little salad with some olive oil)

The rest of the plate: protein (plant protein like beans or nuts, lean meat, fish or a low-fat plain yogurt).

The latest healthy food pyramid recommended is:

At the base of the pyramid: whole grain foods at most meals (oatmeal, whole wheat bread or pasta, brown rice) and plant oils with healthy unsaturated fats like olive and canola oil.

A little higher on the pyramid: vegetables to be eaten in abundance and fruits to be eaten 3 or 4 times per day.

Then fish, chicken or turkey, eggs 0 to twice a day.

Then nuts and legumes 1 to 3 times per day.

Then higher on the pyramid: non-fat dairy and calcium supplements once or twice a day.

At the top: red meat and butter to be used sparingly.

White rice, white bread, potatoes, white pasta, sodas and sweets to be used sparingly.

Alcohol in moderation: not more than one drink per day for women, not more than two drinks per day for men..

It is important to eat at regular hours, at least 3 times a day. You can add 2 healthy snacks in between. If you eat only once a day, you'll send a message to your brain saying that you are in a starving situation and your body will try to store all your calories in fat. This is how people gain weight. If you eat small quantities of healthy food every 3 hours or so, 3 to 5 times a day, everyday at the same time, your body will know that you are not starving and that there is no need to store calories.

If you tend to gain weight, make sure you eat less calories each time you eat but still eat 3 to 5 times a day. You can still eat large quantities of very low calorie foods like lettuce, spinach, thyme, rosemary, basil, oregano, Tarragon, radish, tomatoes, peppers, cucumbers, mushrooms, steamed green beans, broccoli, cauliflower or zucchinis. The important thing is to appreciate them with no dressing or only olive oil and vinegar and no dip or only low fat plain yogurt. Add to this a healthy protein like a lean meat, fish, egg, or vegetable protein like tofu and you have a great meal.

There are a lot of different diets out there: Atkins diet, South Beach diet, Zone diet, Ornish diet, Weight Watchers, Jenny Craig diet. All those diets are good as long as you can stick to them. Find the diet that is the easiest for you to do and stay with it. You will lose weight. Unfortunately if you stop it, you will tend to gain weight again. In the Lyon Diet Heart Study, the Mediterranean diet (with whole grains, fruits, vegetables and fish; limited red meat consumption; butter and cream replaced with canola and olive oils; moderate alcohol) was associated with more than 70% decrease in cardio-vascular mortality and 60% decrease in all cause mortality compared to people on standard recommended post-MI (myocardial infarction) diet.

If you tend to lose weight, eat more calories at least 3 or 4 times a day.

Try to eat mostly simple foods like fruits, salads and vegetables. Try to eat foods that are not processed or processed very little. Look at all the ingredients in all the things you buy. Stay away from processed foods that contain any kind of sugar like glucose, sucrose, cane juice, maple syrup, high fructose corn syrup, honey or any other sugar. If you buy beef, make sure it has only been grass fed.

In general, fast foods like hamburgers, pizzas, fried foods and chips are loaded with bad fats and salt. They are detrimental for your health and should be consumed as sparingly as possible.

Fresh garlic is a very healthy spice which stimulates the immune system and will help you fight bacteria, viruses and fungi. It will also help decrease your bad (LDL) cholesterol and blood pressure and will have an anti-platelet effect (will make your blood thinner). It could possibly help fight cancer.

Turmoric is an anti-inflammatory spice which is full of antioxidants.

Green tea is also rich in anti-oxidants and could have a very good influence on your heart and blood pressure.

Dark chocolate will improve your mood since it gives endorphins and serotonin boosts. It also decreases the bad (LDL) cholesterol and decreases blood pressure. It is wonderful for heart and arteries in general in moderate quantities (not more than 7 ounces per week).

A lot of people come to see me because they are fatigued. As soon as I start them on a "very low sugar diet", they feel much better. It is amazing how much energy digesting sugar can take away from you. Try the "very low sugar diet" yourself and you'll be amazed by the results.

Foods for diabetic patients

One afternoon, a new patient came to see me. She had made an appointment because she felt something was wrong with her. T. was an overweight 43 year old woman who was tired all the time. She was eating sweets and cookies every day at work since they were readily available on her desk. She was thirsty all the time and drinking lots of fruit juices plus soft drinks. The more juices she was drinking the thirstier she was. She was also urinating very often. She indeed didn't look good. A simple blood test made the diagnosis: She had diabetes. I had to change her diet and put her on a very low sugar diet. This is what I told her:

Eat 5 small meals per day and only low glycemic index foods.

Glycemic index measures how quickly your body breaks down sugars. The faster the sugars are broken down in your digestive system, the faster your blood sugar and triglyceride levels will raise and the higher your insulin level will have to be to digest those sugars. Then the faster your blood sugar will drop, the sooner it will drop lower than normal which will make you very hungry again. As you may now understand, this is a vicious cycle.

So, you need to avoid foods that have a high glycemic index such as:

Vegetables: Parsnips, baked potatoes, pumpkin, beets.

Fruits: Watermelon, pineapple, cantaloupe, raisins, dried fruits, mangos, bananas.

Dairy: Ice cream, frozen yogurt.

Cereals which are high in sugar.

Grains: Pretzels, waffles, bagels, instant rice, couscous, crackers, white and wheat bread, hamburger buns, vanilla wafers, croissants.

Other foods: French fries, pizzas, hotdogs, pancakes, scones, dates, doughnuts, muffins, candies, cakes, cookies, tofu frozen desserts, jams and jellies.

<u>You can eat low glycemic index foods such as</u>:

Whole grains but remember that grinding whole wheat until very fine increase its glycemic index.

Vegetables: Lettuce, spinach, kale, aromatic herbs, tomatoes, bell peppers, celery, broccoli, cauliflower, cabbage, green beans, eggplants, yellow squash, zucchini, radishes, asparagus, onions, garlic.

Fruits: Cherries, berries, pears, apples, peaches, plums, oranges and grapefruits (but remember that grapefruits and grapefruit juice can make a lot of conventional medications inactive).

Dairy: plain yogurt, milk.

Legumes: Soy beans, lentils, peas, pinto, kidney or black beans, chickpeas.

Other foods: nuts, olives and dark chocolate.

It is best to eat organic fruits, salads, vegetables, whole grain breads, nuts. You can add fish and meat as long as the meat is as lean as possible. If you eat red meat, eat it in small portions only. You can eat bigger portions of white meats. Eggs are good in small quantities since they are a good source of protein and vitamins.

As for fish, it is recommended since it brings good protein and healthy fats. Avoid large and frequent quantities of the following fish that have a higher concentration of heavy metals like mercury: Shark, swordfish, king mackerel, orange roughy, fresh tuna and tilefish.

One week after starting this very low sugar diet, T's blood sugar was almost in the normal range and she was feeling much better. One month later, she was transformed. She had lost 10 lbs, was eating well, exercising every day, had a lot of energy again and her blood sugar was completely back to normal. What a change this very low sugar diet made on her! 6 months later, she had lost 30 lbs and was looking great!

Foods for high cholesterol and triglyceride levels

S. was a 52 year old man who was the CEO of his company. He was working long hours and eating out every day. Since he had to work long hours, he was eating fast foods when he was by himself and having a lot of business lunches and dinners when he was with customers. As we did his medical check-up, we found that he had a high triglycerides level and high total cholesterol of 273. His good cholesterol was too low to protect him against any heart disease and his bad cholesterol was too high.

Here is what I told him:

Drink less alcohol, no more than one alcoholic drink per day on a weekday, no more than 2 on week-ends.

Eat fewer sweets and starches because your body transforms sweets into triglycerides. Stay away from cookies, cakes and ice cream which contain too much sugar and get your triglyceride level too high.

Eat as little trans-fats as possible. Trans-fats are liquid oils that have been processed (through partial hydrogenation for example) to a partially solid state for a longer shelf life and a higher melting point which makes them attractive for baking. They are not healthy and increase the risk of coronary artery disease.

Eat as little as possible foods high in saturated fats like bacon, hot dogs, pepperoni, pastrami, salami, butter, cheese, sour cream, hamburgers, steaks, chops, ribs, brisket, coconuts, half and half, whole milk, gravies, pizzas. Saturated fat found in animal fat shouldn't comprise more that 10% of daily calories. Eat more mono (olive oil) and polyunsaturated fats (omega-3 and 6).

Eat omega-3 fatty acids- rich foods mostly and be careful with omega-6 fatty acids- rich foods (most seed oils). Metabolites of omega-6 are significantly more inflammatory. They may contribute to allergies, inflammations and cancers. There again, you need a good balance between omega-3s and omega-6s. This means not too much corn oil which has 46 times more omega-6s than omega-3s. As for the other oils, sunflower oil and peanut oil contain no omega-3s; Cotton seed and grape seed oil contain almost no omega-3s. Canola oil contains twice as much omega-6 as omega-3s. This is very acceptable. The best oil is olive oil rich in monounsaturated fat.

Omega-3 fatty acids are mostly EPA (Eicosapentaenoic acid), DHA (Docosahexaenoic acid) and ALA (Alpha linolenic acid) which are found in Flax seeds, eggs, milk, cheeses and meats from grass-fed animals, kelp, perilla seeds, krill (plankton) and fish that eat plankton and algae (wild salmon for example is much richer in omega-3 than farmed raised salmon because it feeds on plankton and algae). They help maintain a healthy heart and circulation and are essential for memory, mood and cognitive functions.

Eat at least 5 servings of low glycemic index fruits and vegetables per day (see list of low glycemic index foods in the "food for diabetic patient" chapter).

Do 30 minutes of physical exercise per day.

S. did really good, changed his diet completely following my guidelines and started walking 45 minutes per day. Within 3 months, his triglycerides and cholesterol went back to normal and he started feeling like a 30 year old again.

Foods against gout

P. was a 61 year old man who had gout attacks at least once a month. His right toe would become so painfully swollen that he couldn't put his shoe on for at least 2 days per month. He was miserable:

I told him to stay away from foods that contain a lot of uric acid (foods that contain Purines).

Foods highest in Purines (150 to 825 mg/100 gm):

Anchovies (363 mg/ 100 gm), sardines, scallops, herring,

Kidney, brain, game meats, gravies, liver.

Foods high in Purines (50 to 150 mg/ 100 gm):

All fish, shellfish, crab, lobster, shrimp, oysters.

Veal, pork, lamb, beef, chicken, duck, turkey meat, meat soups and broths.

Asparagus, cauliflower, mushrooms, spinach.

Legumes, beans, lentils, green peas.

Oatmeal, wheat germ and bran, whole grain breads and cereals.

Are also very rich in Purines: Yeast, beer and wine.

The foods he could eat are the ones that have the lowest amount of Purines:

Coffee, tea, sodas.

Breads and cereals except whole grain.

Cheese, milk, nuts.

Fruits and fruit juices.

Vegetables except those listed above.

Gelatin.

Eggs.

Sugar, syrups, sweets.

Foods to decrease high blood pressure.

M. was 62 years old and had started to have mildly elevated blood pressure 6 months prior. She had only occasional headaches but most often, she had no symptoms.

I told her to eat a little bit of dark chocolate every day for a total amount of 5 oz per week and to drink one or two cups of Hibiscus flower infusion per day.

I told her to avoid high-sodium foods: Leading scientific and governmental agencies advice limiting sodium intake to 2400 mg or less daily. Unfortunately, only 20% of the population meets that objective. In the US diet, 77% of sodium comes from processed and restaurant foods and only 12% occur naturally in foods. Many processed foods contain 1000 mg of sodium or more per serving while a typical restaurant meal contain 2300 to 4600 mg of sodium. Since M. was eating a lot of processed foods and restaurant foods, 2400 mg of sodium was very quickly reached.

For example:

In one biscuit there is 460 to 590 mg of sodium.

In one ounce of American cheese: 290 to 440 mg of sodium.

In one package of Frozen fried chicken dinners: 900 to 2160 mg of sodium.

In one link of hot dog: 420 to 680 mg of sodium.

In 2 tablespoons of salad dressing: 150 to 500 mg of sodium.

In 2 tablespoons of soy sauce: 1840 to 2520 mg of sodium.

In one cup of cream of tomato soup: 340 to 1900 mg of sodium.

As for restaurant food:

In one order of cheese fries with ranch dressing: 4890 mg of sodium.

In one salted bagel: 4520 mg of sodium.

In one order of shrimp with garlic sauce: 2950 mg of sodium.

In one order of fried rice: 2680 mg of sodium.

In one order of Buffalo wings with cheese dressing: 2460 mg of sodium.

In one order of spaghetti with sausage: 2440 mg of sodium.

In one order of lasagna: 2000 mg of sodium.

In one large slice of Combination Pizza: 1580 mg of sodium.

In one Caesar salad: 830 to 1380 mg of sodium.

In one small cheeseburger: 740 to 810 mg of sodium.

In order to eat less than 2400 mg of sodium daily, I told M. to stay away from:

Cured meats: Ham, bacon, sausage, pastrami, hot dogs, smoked fish and meats, lunch meats.

Pickles, olives, cheeses.

Canned goods: soups, vegetables, meats, tuna.

Salted snack foods: chips, salted nuts, crackers.

Baked goods containing baking powder: pancakes, cookies, cakes, pies, biscuits.

Sauces: Ketchup, mustard, soy sauce, Worcestershire sauce, BBQ sauce, salad dressings.

Seasoning: onion salt, garlic salt, celery salt, monosodium glutamate (MSG), bouillon, seasoned salt.

Since she was a little overweight, I told her to decrease her amount of daily calories in order to lose the 10 extra lbs she was carrying.

With this diet, her blood pressure decreased. I still gave her a medication to get her blood pressure completely in the normal range but the low salt diet definitely helped a lot.

Foods to avoid in kidney failure

J. was a 42 year old very nice man who had food poisoning one day. He had a lot of diarrhea and nausea for 3 days and then his kidneys stopped functioning well. He continued being nauseous and having abdominal pain. I treated his food poisoning and he got well again but his kidneys never fully recuperated their function. They had trouble eliminating potassium, phosphorus and uric acid. He was in kidney failure.

I told him to avoid foods that are high in potassium:

High potassium fruits: Apricots, avocados, bananas, cantaloupe, dates, dried fruits, figs, honeydew, mango, nectarine, orange, papaya, plums, prunes, raisins, rhubarb.

High potassium vegetables: Artichokes, beans, broccoli, Brussels sprouts, celery, endive, escarole, greens, kale, lentils, legumes, lima beans, mushrooms, parsnips, potatoes, tomatoes, sweet potatoes.

High potassium other foods: Bran, coffee, chocolate, coconut, molasses, granola, milk, nuts, seeds, tea

<u>I told him to eat foods that are low in potassium:</u>

Low potassium fruits: Apples, blackberries, blueberries, boysenberries, cherries, cranberries, grapes, mandarin oranges, pears, pineapple, raspberries, strawberries, tangerines, watermelon.

Low potassium vegetables: Alfalfa sprouts, asparagus, green beans, bean sprouts, beets, cabbage, carrots, cauliflower, corn, cucumber, eggplant, lettuce, okra, onions, parsley, peas, radish, rutabagas, summer squash, zucchini.

Low potassium other foods: Rice, noodles, breads, cereals, cakes and cookies.

<u>I also told him to stay away from high phosphorus foods like:</u>

High phosphorus beverages: beer, ale, colas, drinks made with milk and cocoa.

High phosphorus protein foods: oysters, crawfish, sardines, animal liver.

High phosphorus vegetables: artichokes, dried beans, broccolis, Brussels sprouts, butternut squash.

Other high phosphorus foods: nuts, seeds, wheat germ, whole grain products, brewer's yeast, peanut butter, milk, cheeses, cottage cheese, ice creams, yogurts, pudding.

I also told him to stay away from all medications that contained a non-steroidal anti-inflammatory like Ibuprofen or Aspirin for example which can be kidney toxic.

Foods rich in Zinc, Magnesium and Selenium

S. was a 16 year old young lady who came to me accompanied by her mother because she was always tired. She was getting sick all the time and had frequent diarrhea. When I examined her, I found a lot of white spots on her fingernails. This made me diagnose a lack of <u>Zinc</u>. I told her to eat more foods that are rich in Zinc such as seeds, soybean products, potatoes, legumes, wheat germs, nuts and red meats. I also prescribed her Zinc supplements. Within 3 months her fatigue resolved and she stopped being sick all the time. When I examined her 8 months later, the white spots on her fingernails had disappeared.

Other people are deficient in <u>Magnesium</u> which can give them muscle spasms, hyperirritability, cardiac arrythmias, fatigue, vertigo. You can find Magnesium in seeds especially pumpkin, soybean products, potatoes, legumes, whole grains, nuts and fresh vegetables.

As for <u>Selenium</u>, it gets incorporated into selenoproteins which are very important antioxidants. They help prevent cellular damage from free radicals. One of the most concentrated food source of Selenium is Brazil nuts. They can contain 70 to 90 micrograms of Selenium per nut. Since we need 100 to 200 microgram of Selenium per day, eating one or two Brazil nuts per day could bring our body a perfect amount of Selenium.

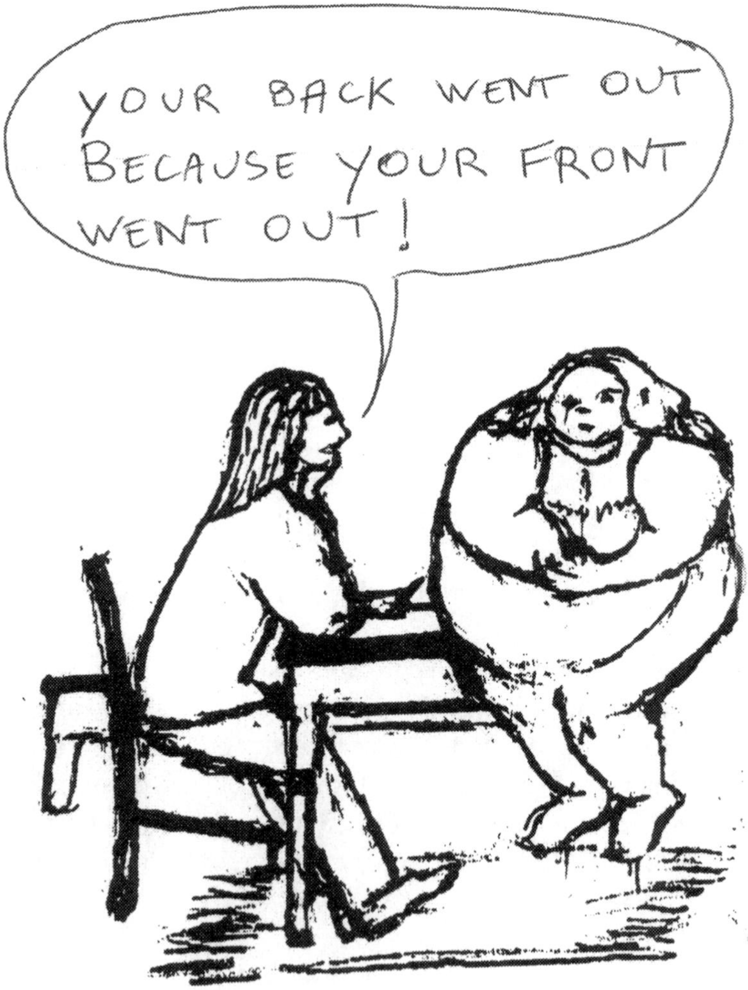
YOUR BACK WENT OUT BECAUSE YOUR FRONT WENT OUT!

Chapter 5
Beverages

Choose the right beverage

"Gluttony is an emotional escape, a sign something is eating us."

Peter De Vries

Just in case you are still wondering, what the right beverage is.... It is WATER! Your body needs water to survive.

One and a half quart of water per day is optimal for most people. If you live in a hot climate, exercise a lot or have a fever, you need even more water. If you don't drink enough, you'll get dehydrated.

How do you know that you are dehydrated? You could be dehydrated if you have: a dry sticky mouth, thirst, muscle weakness, tiredness, sleepiness during the day, headaches, dizziness, lightheadedness and/ or if you stay more than 8 hours without urination and you only have a small amount of dark urine. You could be very dehydrated if you start having a rapid heart rate, low blood pressure and even a fever.

One and a half quart of water per day will help wash out all the toxins, keep your bladder clean and keep your kidneys functioning well. Here again you need the right balance. Can too much water kill you? Yes indeed it can. But it needs to be an enormous amount like more than 10 quarts in a short time. This can happen at water drinking contests where people are challenged to drink as many gallons of water as possible in a few minutes. The concentration of sodium in the serum, around the cells in general and around the brain cells in particular will decrease so much that in order to balance that, water will enter in the brain cells and make them explode. This can be fatal. Do not participate in water drinking contests!

Tap water is as good as bottled water in the United States and Europe. In other countries, don't take the risk of drinking contaminated by bacteria or parasites tap water. In Africa and Mexico, only drink bottled, chlorinated or boiled water. Do not put ice in your drinks unless you know for sure that the ice was made from bottled, chlorinated or boiled water.

Other than water, the best drink is green tea which is full of very healthy antioxidants. It should be drunk without sugar or cream.

Coffee will help you digest and will give you a boost of energy but it shouldn't be drunk in excessive amounts. Again, you need the right balance. Some people do not drink water at all. They drink coffee the whole day. This is too much! Too much coffee could give you palpitations, diarrhea, high blood pressure and insomnia. Do not put sugar in your coffee or cream.

Milk is a great source of Calcium. It is a perfect drink for children in addition to water. Drink low-fat or non-fat milk. But be careful, some children and adults are lactose intolerant. Sometimes, the symptoms of lactose intolerance are subtle: gas, diarrhea, abdominal discomfort. If you have those symptoms, stop all milk products and you might get spectacularly better. You can substitute milk with soy milk which is a wonderful alternative as long as it is unsweetened.

Fruit juices are full of vitamins but only drink the juices that are made with pure fruit and have no sugar added. It is best to just eat the whole fruit which is full of very healthy fiber. Try eating at least 3 servings of fresh fruit per day.

Alcohol can be beneficial as long as it is used in moderation: One glass of wine with dinner will bring good antioxidants. Again, the key word here is moderation. Too much wine or other alcohol could give liver disease.. Do not drink alcohol and drive! You might become responsible for a car accident. Do not drink more than 2 alcoholic drinks per day if you are a man, one alcoholic drink per day if you are a woman! If you think that one alcoholic drink is a whole bottle of wine, think again! One alcoholic drink is for example one glass of wine.

Stay away from regular (non-diet) soft drinks, they contain too much sugar and they contain phosphoric acid which competes with the calcium you are ingesting. It prevents it to be absorbed and will make your bones weaker. A lot of children are obese in our country. Part of this is due to the sodas they drink. One extra large soda bottle per day could make them gain over 20 lbs per year and make them more prone to bone fractures. Occasionally, if you engage in strenuous physical activity, you need to replenish water, salt and sugar in which case Gatorade and other similar drinks are good to drink during exercise and right afterwards.

The big trend now is to buy energy drinks. I do not recommend them unless you are engaging regularly in strenuous physical exercise. They have a long list of ingredients and a lot of those ingredients are not healthy starting with some kind of sugar.

One kind of sugar that is used more and more often is Sorbitol in its pure form or in a form of Polysorbate. Some people are Sorbitol intolerant. Sorbitol will give them abdominal discomfort and bloating. You need to look at all the ingredients of everything you are buying. The longer the list, the more risks there are that something will not agree with your body. Try to stick to simple drinks.

As for vitamins and vitamin waters, my take on them is that as long as you eat fresh fruits, nuts, salads and vegetables every day and as long as you eat fish and white meat from time to time, you have all the vitamins your body needs. You don't need extra ones. Extra vitamins will not make you live longer. They might even shorten your life.

Chapter 6
Breathe good quality air

"Fresh air impoverishes the doctor."

Danish proverb

The air we breathe is made of 20.95% oxygen, 78% nitrogen, 1% water vapor and trace amounts of other gases. Through photosynthesis, trees and other plants absorb carbon dioxide and release oxygen into the atmosphere.

Clean air is important for good health. Make sure you live and work in an area that has a lot of trees and is not polluted. Try not to live too close to a heavily trafficked road, a nuclear plant or a chemical factory.

If you are driving in rush hour traffic, you are exposed to the exhausts of other cars. If your air vents are open, you might be inhaling brake dust, carbon monoxide and diesel fumes. Make sure you have good air filters or close air vents before and during bumper to bumper travel. Do not make your car engine run in a closed garage.

Wear a mask covering your nose and mouth while doing construction work like sanding, wood work or concrete work.

Make sure you don't have a faulty furnace or carozene heater. Make sure you have an exhaust above your gas stove and that the smoke sensors in your house are working properly. Poisoning by carbon monoxide may occur after exposure to automobile exhaust, smoke inhalation in a fire for example or improperly vented gas heater or other appliance. You might think you will see the gas or smell it. Well, in reality, you won't because carbon monoxide is colorless and odorless. The first symptoms of carbon monoxide poisoning include headaches, dizziness, abdominal pain and nausea. With more advanced intoxication come confusion, shortness of breath, syncope and seizures, then coma and death. The specific treatment is highly concentrated oxygen.

Do not breathe in the face of somebody coughing in front of you. Politely, turn your face away to breathe. If you, yourself are coughing, cover your mouth when coughing. You do catch germs by breathing contaminated air. You also catch germs by touching contaminated handrails, doorknobs or countertops with your hands and then putting your fingers in your nose. Make sure you wash your hands with soap and water frequently. If it is too late and you shook the hand of several flu-sick people then stuck your fingers in your nose, put some hydrogen peroxide on a Q-tip and paint the inside of your nostrils with it. This will hopefully prevent the germs from infecting you.

When the air is too dry, use a humidifier and make sure you drink enough water. On airplanes for example, the air is extremely dry and you can benefit from drinking one glass of water every hour or so.

At high altitudes, oxygen gets rarer. You could get short of breath and tired easily. Your lungs will need a few days to adjust to high altitude.

Once you are inhaling good quality air, make sure you are inhaling deeply, opening all the alveoli in your lungs. Make sure you are exhaling deeply getting all the carbon dioxide out of your alveoli.

When we exert ourselves, we tend to breathe deeply but when we are stressed out or working at our computer most of the day, we tend to breathe in a shallow way. A lot of alveoli only fill up part way with oxygen.

A good meditation technique is to take a few minutes every morning to focus only on your breathing. If a thought comes to mind, send it away. Visualize all your alveoli opening and filling up with pink clean oxygen-charged air when inhaling. Then, visualize all your alveoli getting rid of dark grey carbon dioxide-charged air when exhaling. Breathe deeply this way at least 5 times in a row when waking up in the morning or when you feel stressed out. This will make you feel immediately better and will make every cell in your body function better.

Chris Elisabeth Gilbert, M.D., Ph.D.

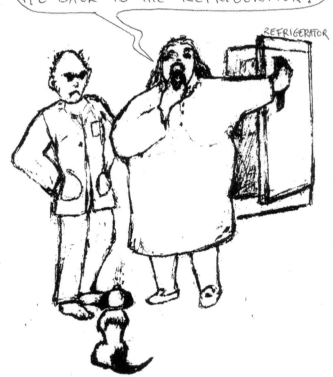

Chapter 7
Sleep

"A good laugh and a good sleep are best cures
in the doctor's book."

Irish proverb

A third of your life is spent sleeping. So, it is important that this third of your life is spent comfortably. Make sure you have the right mattress which should be firm and flat. If your mattress has a big hole in it – which for example has the shape of your bottom – get rid of it and buy a new mattress.

Try going to bed and getting up at the same time every day. Make sure you get enough sleep for your body. Some people only need 5 hours of sleep per night. Others need 9 hours. Determine what your body needs and give it the right amount every night.

During sleep, the right amount of hormones is being secreted, your immune system gets organized and your brain neurons get connected. Even though it doesn't seem so, your body is working during the time you sleep and this work is indispensable for a healthy life.

Read a book or listen to music before bedtime.

Avoid watching TV before sleep and avoid eating a very heavy meal just before bedtime.

Avoid drinking coffee and other caffeinated drinks. Avoid taking Vitamin C in the evening. They might prevent you from falling asleep.

If you have trouble sleeping, go for a walk in the evening! Have sex at bedtime! You'll then have a great night sleep.

If you are in a noisy environment, use foam earplugs. They are very comfortable and they can make all the difference between a peaceful uninterrupted sleep and being woken up by the snoring of your partner or by noisy neighbors.

When I was a resident in the surgical Intensive Care Unit at Harbor-UCLA, I was on call every other day. I had to work from 6 am to 8 pm at night, was on call the whole night and had to work the following day from 6 am to sometimes 2 pm. That was 32 hours of work in a row. Then I had until 6 am the following day to recuperate then I was on call again. My call nights were so busy that I was lucky if I got 30 minutes of uninterrupted sleep in the 32 hours I was at the hospital. I had to do this every other day. Needless to say that after one month, I was so sleep deprived that I promised myself to always appreciate a night without a pager waking me up every 5 minutes. If you have trouble falling asleep, try staying active most of the day and night. Lie down on your bed only 4 hours – from 2 am to 6 am - 5 nights in a row. Chances are that the 6th night, you'll start sleeping well.

If you have trouble falling asleep, do this exercise at bedtime:

Stretch your right extended leg 3 inches up from the bed, contracting all your right leg muscles, hold it there for 5 seconds, then release and breathe deeply. Do the same thing with your left leg. Then stretch your right arm 2 inches up from the bed, contracting all your right arm muscles and making a tight fist, hold it there for 5 seconds, then release and breathe deeply. Do the same thing with your left arm. Lift your shoulders up towards your head, hold them up for 5 seconds, then release and breathe deeply. Squeeze your shoulders together behind your back for 5 seconds, then release and breathe deeply. Squeeze your buttocks muscles together hold this for 5 seconds, then release and breathe deeply. Inhale as deeply as you can hold it for 5 seconds, then release and breathe deeply. Squeeze your abdominal muscles in hold it for 5 seconds, then release and breathe deeply. Open your mouth as wide as possible hold it for 5 seconds, then release and breathe deeply.

Then, take a few deep breaths; breathe out all the stress by imagining breathing out dark black air. When you breathe in, imagine breathing in pink clean air. As you do this, put all the stress in an imaginary air balloon and when you are done, blow it up in the air far away from you into the sky. Once your stress-loaded hot air balloon is gone from your sight, imagine a dream that you would like to have, something you would like to achieve and actively start your dream. Make up every detail of your dream and before you know it, you will be fast asleep. When I cannot fall asleep, I imagine I am an actress in a movie. I visualize the scene and all the other well-known actors I am with. This makes me so happy that I fall asleep quickly and have wonderful dreams.

Do not concentrate on negative thoughts before falling asleep; always make the active effort to concentrate on positive thoughts, on all the good things that happened during your day, on your hopes for the future and on the things you would like to achieve.

In order to help you, name everything that gave you support in your life. How did you get to today and now? Name the people, the animals, flowers, sceneries, foods, smells and colors that supported you at any time in your life. Feel how huge your support is. With that much support, you can achieve anything and everything you want. Feel how much power you have. This will help you have a restful sleep.

For example, when I have trouble falling asleep, I thank all the support I had and what I still have now: my family, my best friends, my pets, my house which I love and my car which drives beautifully and in which I feel so good. My support system doesn't end there. I get support from my favorite colors turquoise and purple. Everything I buy tends to be either turquoise or purple or the combination of both. For some reason those colors make me feel good. I also get support from my favorite perfumes, from smelling the roses, listening to the birds, eating my favorite foods, going to the beach at least once a week, from the sound of the waves and from breathing in fresh air from the seaside. The list of my support system doesn't end there. I get support from having a healthy heart, lungs, liver and kidneys. I get support from my legs and arms that are working wonderfully without pain. I get support from living in a country where I can buy all the foods I like. I get support from the warmth of the sun and from getting into a hot bath. I get support from the clothes I wear and from my favorite shoes. As you can see the list of my support system is huge and I can still find a lot more. I recommend you to do the same exercise at night if you have trouble falling asleep or if you feel depressed. It will be a tremendous help.

Chapter 8
Physical exercise: Exercise the right way for your body

"Those who think they have no time for bodily exercise will sooner or later have to find time for illness."

Edward Stanley

One golden rule is 10,000 steps per day! Your body needs regular exercise! It was not created for sitting at your computer desk 8 to 12 hours a day without moving. It was created to walk and run.

The worse possible position for your back, the worse possible thing for your arteries is to sit for long hours without moving. Your muscles will tend to atrophy and you'll have severe backache. Your arteries will clog up. You'll be at risk of a heart attack and you might experience pain in your legs when walking.

You need to get your blood flowing. The best way is to exercise every day at least 30 minutes per day (60 minutes is even better) in the morning when getting up but also during the day. Do warm up exercises with stretches before any physical exercise so that you don't pull muscles. Toning of muscles can be achieved by using weights (resistance training) which will boost your metabolism. Women will benefit from using 2 to 3 lbs weights, men will benefit from using

5 or 8 lbs weights. Do push ups and sit ups then go to the gym, lift light weights, go jogging, bicycling, swimming, play tennis or golf. Those have excellent cardiovascular benefits. In your senior years, Tai Chi will be a wonderful exercise which will bring you balance and strengthen your body, mind and spirit.

Do not sit in a chair more that 2 hours in a row without getting up. Every couple of hours, stretch your arms and legs, go for a walk, go up and down the stairs. Find an excuse to get up at least every couple of hours. Make every joint work. When a joint works too little, it might get damaged. On the other hand, do not overstress your joints. If you run on concrete several hours a day every day for example, it could damage your knees. You need to find the right balance for your joints, not too little exercise but not too much either.

When you drive somewhere, park far away from the place you want to go to so that you can get some walking done. 10,000 steps per day is what you need to achieve. When the place you are going to is on the 2nd or 3rd floor, use stairs instead of elevators.

A great tool to use for your back is: hanging from a bar with your hands.

Several of my patients used to complain about lower back pain. They needed to go to the chiropractor "all the time" to "get readjusted" and needed to take anti-inflammatory medications very often. I told them to install a solid bar in one of their doorframe and to start hanging from it with their hands a few seconds once or twice a day. Within a few days, their lower back pain resolved without any chiropractic care or anti-inflammatory medication. I myself have such a bar in my home and I hang from it a few seconds 2 or 3 times a day. It is better to weigh less than 300 lbs to use such a bar. You hold it with 2 hands which you should position about two feet from each other then slowly you lift your legs up in front of you. It stretches your back instantly and readjusts all the vertebrae on the spot. Use the bar shortly after lifting something heavy, after a long car trip or after a long day at work. It gives instantaneous relief but you might want to consult your physician before you do this to make sure it is appropriate for you.

I myself exercise 30 minutes every morning. I start with arms exercises, pulling my arms straight up and down 10 times then I do circles with my arms fully extended 20 times then I do push ups. I lie down on my back and lift 5 lbs weighs up and down 20 times then I do abdominal muscles exercises remaining on my back. I lift my legs up and do 50 bicycle movements without weights and then I attach a 2 lbs weight on each foot and do the same bicycle movements again. I get up and stand on my tip toes going up and down 20 times then I run around my house for 10 minutes. At the end, I hang from my bar. All this gives me a 30 minutes routine everyday to which I add a one hour walk 3 to 4 times a week. This allows me to be in great physical shape the whole week.

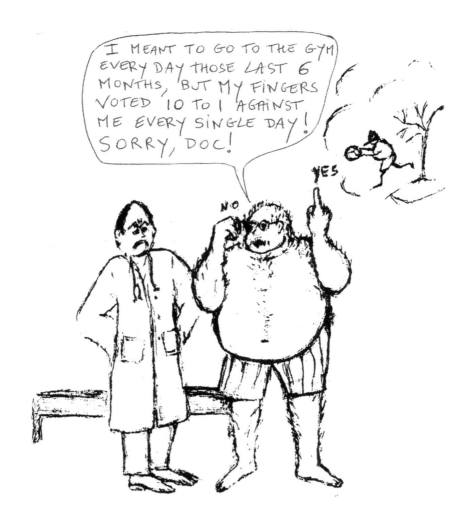

Chapter 9
Stress

"Stress is nothing more than a socially acceptable form of mental illness."

Richard Carlson

What is Stress?

Stress is a physical (for example you miss a step and fall down) or psychological stimulus (for example your boss is giving you 10 new reports to write and they need to be ready by tomorrow!) which tends to disturb the normal physiological equilibrium of the body.

With acute stress, all our protection mechanisms go on high alert. It starts with the brain: Our hypothalamus and pituitary gland secrete hormones to prepare the rest of our body for fighting. Our adrenal glands react to the alert by releasing adrenaline which makes the heart pump faster and the lungs work harder. Our nerve cells release norepinephrine which tenses the muscles and sharpens the senses to prepare for action. Digestion then shuts down. All this is protective and prepares our body to fight.

If acute stress remains a long time, it becomes chronic stress. It can be caused by constant emotional pressure that we can't control.

For example: Most of you probably have kids; you need to get up early in the morning, get the children ready for the day then go to work and put in your 8 to 10 hours of work for the day, then, do grocery shopping, pick up your kids from school, take them to soccer practice then pick them up again, spend some time with them, clean the house, prepare meals, do dishes, be sexual with your spouse.... Without counting that last phone call from your Mom who seems to have the flu and needs help. You are starting to be stressed out!

What are some of the symptoms of Stress?

They can vary depending on the individual: Increase in heart rate, respiration rate and blood pressure, headaches, constipation, worsening of asthma, nausea, diarrhea, abdominal pain and sexual difficulties.

It can create an increased secretion of Cortisol (hormone secreted by your adrenal glands) which can give high blood sugar, high blood pressure, gastric pain, gastric ulcer and weaker bones. Why weaker bones? Because your guts won't absorb much calcium any more nor potassium! The priority is given to sodium and water which will cause high blood pressure.

Other symptoms of stress are increased susceptibility to infections, acne, insomnia, irritability, women will not have their period any more or it will skip a month.

Those women might then decide to eat more, especially those delicious sweets that calm them down. Not a good choice because they are going to gain weight...

Burger: 490 Cal, French Fries: 220 Cal, Regular Soda: 144 Cal. Altogether 854 Cal.

In order to eliminate those calories, they need to walk up and down the stairs for one hour.

At home, your children are smarter than you think they are. They can feel that you are under a lot of stress and therefore will demand more attention. The more stressed out you are, the more attention your children will require and the more difficult they will be to raise. This will make you even more stressed out...

By the way, when a woman is pregnant, she thinks that the embryo in her uterus doesn't feel her stress. Wrong!

The more stressed out she is during pregnancy, the more difficult and demanding the baby will be when he or she is born. This baby will then be a difficult infant and a stressed out adult like mom.

The more unhealthy foods she eats during her pregnancy, the more unhealthy foods her child will be uncontrollably drawn to in the future.

And it is not the end of the possible damage...

Some people have atherosclerosis with deposit of fatty material along the coronary arteries which are the arteries bringing oxygen to the heart. With stress, their liver will secrete a chemical called C-Reactive Protein (CRP). This CRP will create inflammation around the deposits of fatty material. Over time, the plaque which was in a major artery will then detach, become free floating and migrate downstream to completely block the blood from flowing which could create a heart attack.

Let us talk about another disease which is cancer: People who are relaxed and happy will fight their cancer better and will live a longer time than people who are depressed and stressed out. At Stanford, they did a study on metastatic breast cancer patients. They measured a stress indicator: Their Cortisol level! The women who had the highest levels of Cortisol (higher stress) had survival rates a year and a half shorter then women with the lowest Cortisol (lower stress) level.

Try to avoid what causes stress: Choose a work that is not too stressful and if stress at work is sometimes unavoidable, try to avoid stress at home. Be nice to your spouse. Be understanding yet firm with your children. Watch your step when you walk or run and be very careful driving.

Try not to eat too much. You'll find that eating can reduce stress but this comes at a very high price of obesity, joint pain, high cholesterol or triglycerides and much more.

Try not to drink too much alcohol. Yes, alcohol reduces stress but you risk becoming dependent on it. Women, do not have more than one drink per day. Men, do not have more than 2 drinks per day. Otherwise you are at risk of liver damage.

Try not to drink too much coffee and don't smoke.

Make sure you have enough sleep at night (see Chapter on Sleep). Lack of sleep will make you more sensitive to stress.

Decrease your stress by getting some physical exercise regularly. Go for a walk, a run or go to the gym 4 times a week (see Chapter on Physical exercise). Start yoga, pilates, meditation or tai-chi. Spend 30 minutes per day working on your hobby. Have regular sex with your partner and take the time to enjoy it.

Do the maximum you can to decrease your everyday stress.

Chapter 10
Find your Passion in Life

"Passion is universal humanity; without it, religion, history, romance and art would be useless."

Honore de Balzac

What do you enjoy doing? What makes you vibrate? What could you do for the rest of your life without getting bored or tired?

My 2 passions in life are practicing medicine and acting. If I spend too much time doing only one of them, I become weaker and get sick. After a few weeks of seeing patients in my private practice, I need to be on a TV show as an actress and also very often as a medical adviser. This gives me a real boost of energy. After several days on a TV show working long hours, I am really happy to get back to my private practice. The balance between TV shows and my private practice is my passion in life.

Everybody has a different passion. Every person was born with a special unique gift, something he or she loves to do and is good at. When we were a child, that gift was obvious but it sometimes disappeared under parents or peer pressure. It is now time to find it again and make it blossom. Spend at least 15 minutes per day trying to find it and then spend at least 15 minutes per day pursuing it.

S. was working in a company that required her to be on call 24/7. She hated her job which was making her terribly stressed out. She had no time to exercise and was eating in fast food restaurants all the time. She started gaining weight and 80 additional lbs later, her back started hurting tremendously. That's when she came to my office. She told me that her dream had always been to create her own home health company. She started taking classes on owning your own business. A few months later, she was able to quit her job to become CEO of her own company. She started exercising and stopped all junk foods. 6 months later, I could barely recognize her. She was looking so good and so healthy, fit and energetic. She had a big smile on her face. She had lost 60 lbs, was exercising every day and had no more backache. Her new company was thriving.

If we are forced to do something we hate, our immune system will get weaker, our hormones won't be secreted as perfectly and we'll get sick faster. On the other hand, it is amazing to witness what happens in our brain and in the rest of our body when we do something we love: Our immune system gets stronger; every single one of our cells works better; we have more energy than ever; we tend to be more productive and successful.

Make sure you are spending at least 15 minutes per day or 2 hours per week doing something you really enjoy!

Chapter 11
Spend quality time by yourself

"We must be our own before we can be another's."

Ralph Waldo Emerson

Spending time alone can be scary for some people but when it is done the right way, it is quite wonderful. It is actually necessary for rebalancing. After a hard day at the office and after spending time in traffic coming back home, your brain could be very tired. If you don't spend time by yourself getting back in balance, you might push your body too hard and hurt it.

Most men need at least 15 to 30 minutes of quiet time when coming back home after a hard day at work. Most wives and children should learn to respect that. For most women however, quiet time alone isn't enough. They can benefit greatly from a meditation technique for rebalancing. Here is one example of de-stressing exercise.

Spend at least 10 minutes per day doing the following:

Sit comfortably, close your eyes and listen to your breathing. Breathe in visualizing clean positive energy going up from your belly to your navel then to your sternum to your throat to your forehead to the top of your head. Hold your breath a few seconds then breathe out visualizing your black negative energy going down from the top of your head to your forehead to your throat to your sternum to your belly button to your belly and then leaving your body. Continue this exercise for as long as you can and as long as your body needs it. It will rebalance you. Then concentrate on something beautiful like a beautiful flower or scenery and breathe in the beauty inside you. You can also concentrate on a certain smell or a sound that you like (sound of music, sound of a bird, etc…).

Learn to stay alone with nature and gain strength form it. Learn this now as it will come in very handy in the future when you'll go through hard times. Living life is like surfing the waves. If you learn how to surf small waves, it will be easier to surf big waves in the future. Unfortunately, chances are you will be faced with very big waves. People that are very dear to you will disappear and you, yourself might face hardships either financial or physical. Big waves might smash you and destroy you if you don't learn how to surf them.

Your alone time will allow you to be in touch with your 6 boards. This will add a new dimension to your life.

I went to Christine Price's workshop in Big Sur in 2007. She talked about life's 5 boards: the Surfboard, the keyboard, the boardroom, the switchboard, the circuit board. I would add a 6th one: the dashboard. This made a lot of sense for my own life and it probably does for most people. Here are the 6 boards and the way I experienced them for myself:

My surfboard: Living my life is like surfing the ocean. Sometimes I am faced with small waves and I surf them well, sometimes I am faced with big waves and I get smashed. I get up and I learn how to surf them. I learn how to surf bigger and bigger waves. The better surfer I am, the easier life becomes for me. When my father died, it was a very high wave. I spent a lot of time with him, helping him as much as I could. I had to spend a lot of alone time too. I took energy from the beauty of the ocean, the birds and the flowers. I meditated on my breathing. I surfed the wave of loss as best as I could. I didn't think I could surf any bigger wave then my wonderful husband died. That's when I really got smashed and fell hard. I didn't think I could get back up and surf again but I did. I surfed the wave of loss and intense deep grief and pain as best as I could. Sometimes, we try to stop the waves but it takes a lot of energy to control the universe. It takes a lot of our vitality. Unfortunately, there are more and more waves coming. If all we use our energy for, is trying to control the waves, we'll quickly get very tired. We'll have a lot of work trying to make the ocean flat and at the end, we won't succeed. It is much better to learn how to surf the waves. For this, we need to use our breath. We need to say yes to the experience whatever it is.

My dashboard: Every day, I need to look at my dashboard: Is there enough gas for the day, enough oil, water? Am I going too fast or too slow? Is my engine overheating? Am I drinking enough water, eating the right food, exercising enough, spending enough time by myself, with friends and family? My dashboard shows: "Today you are in red, your engine is overheating, you'll need to rest more this week-end" or "Today you didn't drink enough water" or "you ate too much". I look at my dashboard and fix the problem immediately. If I don't pay attention to my dashboard, my engine might blow up and it could be a disaster.

My keyboard: There are different notes in me that need to be expressed. There is Chris the romantic, the happy Chris, the sad Chris, the angry Chris, the sexual Chris, the funny Chris, the loving Chris, the witty Chris, the frustrated Chris, the fulfilled Chris, Chris the singer, Chris the actress, Chris the writer, Chris the physician. All my keys can be very intense. I am usually only playing the main notes, the ones I am used to, the ones everybody else is used to. The other ones are there though and when they are allowed to come out, I become this human being full of colors and music. I love all my notes on my keyboard. They make me feel full. Everybody has a similar yet different keyboard. We are born as a piano with a lot of keys. Some keys we were or are forbidden to play, some other keys, we were or are forced to play. Some keys, we are very much in touch with, they are our established resources. Some other keys are there but we don't want those tones. We are aware of them but we try to suppress them. Some keys, we really like in other people but we don't think we have them in us. Learning how to play on our keyboard is learning how to make beautiful music, learning how to live an intense beautiful life.

My switchboard: I have several parts of me that need to be expressed. Acting is my hobby and sometimes the actress in me needs to come out and do a play or be on a TV show. Other times the serious physician in me needs to come out. I also love when the funny, witty and sexy me comes into play. Using my switchboard allows the different parts of me to express themselves as they need to.

My boardroom: When I need to make an important decision, I need to call in all the parts of myself in my boardroom. This is what happened when I left Paris, France where I grew up. Chris the actress wanted to live near Hollywood, Dr. Chris the physician wanted to live in the United States, Chris the romantic woman wanted to marry an American man (they are so romantic and respectful!), Chris the hay fever child wanted to live at the seaside, Chris the always too cold lady wanted to live in a warm country. All of them got together, had a board meeting and they all agreed that Los Angeles would be perfect for all of them. That is how I moved to Los Angeles. You need to have board meetings from time to time and respect the opinions of all the different parts of you. Every different part of you has a piece of the truth. Nobody has the whole truth. Every part needs a little time and a little air (the vulnerable, the violent, etc...). Every part needs to be heard. It doesn't need to be in the driver's seat but it needs to be acknowledged. If you don't acknowledge each and every part, you will be unhappy and if you are unhappy, chances are that you will make the people around you unhappy too. Then your body might fail you.

My circuit board: I have a certain electric power that I can sustain. If things get too intense for too long, I'll blow a fuse and will be out of order until I can heal myself and restore my power. On the other hand, if the electricity is not strong enough, my circuit board will not work. There will not be enough power to make my body function. I need to stay aware of this and keep the intensity at a right level.

You too need to be aware of your 6 boards and it will be a great help in your life if you can master them. In your alone time, have a board meeting. Also appreciate the fact that you can breathe freely, that your heart is beating harmoniously, that your hands and feet are moving with no pain, that you can see, hear, smell, touch and taste life to perfection. Knowing your own body and its limits and being able to deal with all your boards harmoniously will boost your health and energy tremendously.

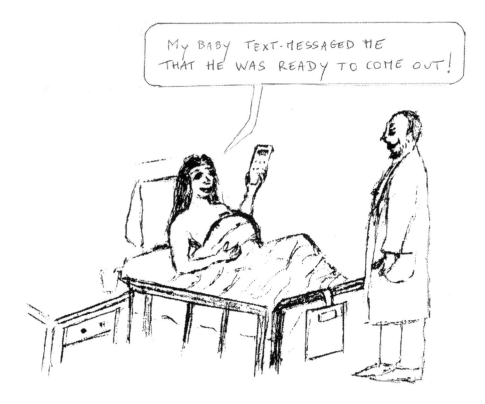

Chapter 12
Find the right mate.

*"Let your love be like the misty rains, coming softly,
but flooding the river."*

Malagasy proverb

Finding the right mate may seem easy but in reality, it isn't.

You think you only need to fall in love and that will be enough to live happily ever after. Well, the reality is very different: Your mate needs to be a compatible person. The key word here is compatible.

You need to be compatible in 7 different levels:

- Spiritually
- Emotionally
- Sexually
- Intellectually
- Financially
- You need to share the same ideas as far as how many children to have and how to raise them.
- You need to share the same ideas as far as where to live, how big a house and land to have, how to decorate the place.

Sharing a hobby is an added bonus.

J. and A. are 23 and 25 years old and are deeply in love with each other and are about to get married. J. doesn't believe in God, likes to have sex every day, doesn't like to buy expensive things and tries to save a lot of money for retirement, doesn't want children and is happy in his small condo. A. on the other hand, is very religious, Catholic going to church every Sunday, only likes to have sex once or twice a month, likes to spend a lot of money on fancy clothes and jewelry, would like to have 3 children and would like to live in a large expensive house. They are deeply in love with each other but is their marriage going to be a happy one? Probably not! They are too incompatible on too many different levels. A marriage would be a disaster. It would take a very heavy toll on their bodies and would probably create diseases.

Unfortunately, we don't learn this at school. We learn how to be successful in business; we don't learn how to have a successful marriage.

Let's talk about something that is not taught in school or by our parents: making love. Making love seems obvious but it really isn't. It's easy for men to have an orgasm. It is not that easy for women. You as a couple need to learn how to use the different ways of touching each other from static touch to moving touch to light squeezing. You need to explore the different methods of kissing each other, kissing that can be applied to any part of the body. Use lipping, tonguing, sucking and blowing kisses. Once inside each other, vary positions, depth, speed, angle of entry and types of movements. Making love is an art which can take time to master. Reading the book "Tantra: the art of conscious loving" by Charles and Caroline Muir published by Mercury House will help you master it in the most beautiful way.

Know that people grow over time and their priorities in life will change. J. in 10 years will be 35 years old and will still want to make love every day or every other day. A. will be 33 years old and will probably have 3 children to take care of. Her priority will be her children and her house. She might not be interested in love making any more. All her time and energy will be used for her children and her part-time work. Then what will J. do?

Know that when you marry somebody, you are also marrying your partner's family and all the benefits and responsibilities that come with it, responsibilities of parents, sisters, brothers and children from previous marriages. Women, make sure you meet your future husband's father and like him because your husband might become just like his father 30 years later. Men, look at your future mother-in-law and know that your future wife might become just like her in another 30 years.

Being with the wrong mate will bring you stress and diseases will come more easily.

Being with the right mate will bring you balance and will help you fight diseases. Making love will make you produce endorphins. Laughing will make your body function better. Having a mate who is your best friend is a wonderful asset for your health.

If you are with the wrong mate and don't have children with him or her yet, leave the relationship! If you have children with him or her already, it is probably too late. Damage will be impossible to avoid. If you leave this mate, your children will be damaged; if you stay, you will be damaged. Children from divorced parents are marked forever. It is an intensely traumatic experience for them. It is chaos. They will have to get familiar with chaos to survive and when it will be time for them to choose a mate, they will choose chaos because it is familiar. How are they supposed to know what a perfect match is? How are they supposed to know what real love is? They don't! Of course, they will tend to choose the wrong mate and they will get divorced too. That's why it is so important to recognize early enough in the relationship that it is the wrong mate for you and to take time to choose the right partner. You need to make sure that he or she will be the right father or mother for your children. Forget about marrying somebody with whom you are passionately in love but with whom you don't feel good on an everyday life.

Try finding a partner with whom you feel incredibly good, at ease, with whom you can laugh and who loves you. Make sure you are compatible spiritually, emotionally, sexually, intellectually, financially, that you share the same ideas as far as how many children to have and how to raise them and that you share the same ideas as far as where to live. This will provide you with happiness, stability and good health. This will show your children what a happy marriage is and as a consequence, they will tend to choose the right partner for them too.

Chapter 13
Spend quality time with family and friends

"Almost every wise saying has an opposite one, no less wise, to balance it."

Santayana - Essays

Let's start with your friends: Contrary to your parents and children whom you cannot choose, you do choose your friends. It is important that you choose the right friends for you, the ones that support you, and the ones that have a positive energy. Some people have friends that make them feel bad and have a negative energy. Getting rid of those friends might be the right thing to do. It is important that you feel good with friends, that you do fun relaxing activities together, share hobbies and that you have constructive talks with them. This will have a positive impact on your health.

Let's talk about spirituality. Deep inside, what is your faith? Once you know what it really is, attend your church, synagogue or mosque on a regular basis. It will decrease your stress and will provide a peaceful environment for a healthier lifestyle away from negative influences like alcohol and drugs. It will help you grow spiritually. It will provide strength and positive meaning to your life.

Now, let's talk about your parents. Unfortunately, you didn't choose them. Some people were lucky enough to have good parents who gave them a lot of love and support. I am one of those. My parents gave me unconditional love and support and showed me the example of a perfect couple. This made it very easy for me to love them and support them when they needed me.

A lot of people were not that lucky. Some people never got unconditional love. If you don't get along with your parents or if they are evil, don't see them too often. When you see them, just be polite with them. Try to help them as much as you can but don't expect anything in return. If they are not good people, make sure you shield yourself from their negative energy. If you don't, you might get sick.

One of my patients, R. used all her vacation time to help her mother who couldn't care less and treated her very badly. Each time R .came back from seeing her mother, she got sick and it was very difficult for me to put her back on her feet. It put a stain on her relationship with R's husband. When the energy is negative and destructive, stay away from the situation if you can or minimize the amount of time you have to stay.

On the other hand, if you get along well with your parents, make sure you spend quality time with them and make sure you are there for them at the end of their lives. They will be scared and they will need your unconditional love. Being there for them is extremely important. It will bring them the ultimate support they need to leave this world and it will bring you peace for the rest of your own life.

Your children's situation is different yet the same. If you chose to have children, you need to give them the best of you. You need to give them all the love, attention and education you can. You cannot create children and spend all your time working long hours away from them. They need *you, your* presence and *your* time. They need your love and your teachings. They don't need a nanny, they don't need daycare! They need *you*! Their first few years of life are extremely important. They decide of the rest of their life.

My patient J. was never loved by her parents. They never spent time with her. She was always in daycare. Her mother always criticized her when she was there. She was never doing anything right. Her parents had a really bad relationship and ended up getting a divorce when she was 10 years old. The first years of J's life had a disastrous effect on her. To this day- she is now 49 years old- she feels a void in her life. She still thinks she is not doing anything right. She never felt pretty even though she is a very beautiful woman. She chose the wrong husband who beat her up and she is now getting a divorce herself. She is always sick, going from one illness to another. She is never able to appreciate life. The way her parents treated her ruined her whole life. Now that her parents are dead, she still cannot get back on her feet.

Children are very vulnerable even though they seem so strong at times. Depending on how you treat them the first few years of their lives, you will determine the rest of their lives. That's how much power you have! You can make them miserable for the rest of their lives or you can make them happy for the rest of their lives. Pick one!

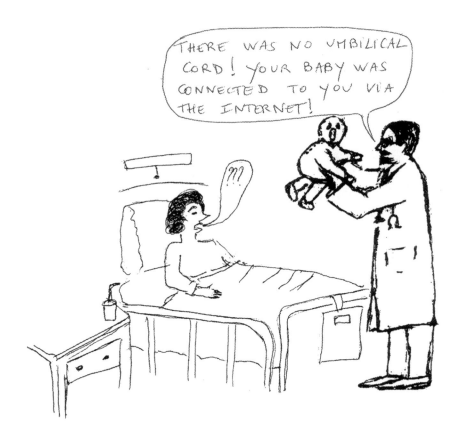

Chapter 14
Appreciate what you have

"The secret of health for both mind and body is not to mourn for the past, not to worry about the future, or not to anticipate troubles, but to live the present moment wisely and earnestly."

Buddha

An optimistic sees a solution to every problem. A pessimist sees a problem with every solution!

You can look at the same situation from two opposite points of view, one is positive and the other is negative. It comes down to: Do you see the glass half full or half empty?

Always look at the positive side of what you have, even if you have very little. Looking at the positive side will boost your immune system, will make you secrete those good endorphins you like and will make you feel wonderful. If you start concentrating on the negative side of what you don't have, your immune system will get weaker and you'll start feeling depressed which will make you even weaker. You'll start spiraling down and you will get sick more and more often.

When I was working in a refugee camp in Sri Lanka in the North of the Island, I had no electricity, no running water, no hot water heater and the food was very simple with mostly rice and chicken. I was the only physician for 27,000 refugees and I was on call 24/7. I was lucky when I could sleep 4 uninterrupted hours without being woken up by an emergency. It was so hot (over 88 degrees at night) that I had to manually fan myself to get to sleep. I used candle light for reading at night. I washed every morning with cold water from a bucket. I was sleep-deprived and missed eating fresh salads, vegetables and fruits. Yet, I tried to only concentrate on what I had. It was very fulfilling to help so many sick people who had even less than what I had. I appreciated my bucket of cold water in the morning; I enjoyed my candle for reading and the leaf I was using as a fan to cool down. I enjoyed eating rice and chicken and was thankful that I wasn't starving and always had drinking water as much as I needed. I was always thankful when I got a good night sleep. I was always thankful to be healthy and strong. I was thankful I had a roof above my head and a bed to come to at night (even though I had to share a small bedroom with 2 other people). I had very little but by appreciating what I had, I remained very happy and physically very strong.

On the other hand, A. a patient of mine came to see me because she was very unhappy. She was living in a big house with a beautiful garden, having hot water and a Jacuzzi, having all the possible delicious food she could eat, all the possible drinks she would like, sleeping without interruption at night and having a great healthy body. Unfortunately, she was not appreciating any of those and was only thinking about the way her boyfriend was criticizing her all the time. This was the only thing in her mind and she was so unhappy that she became severely depressed. She started having backaches and a sore throat all the time. What was my role as her doctor? Give her pain killers and antibiotics? I tried once. Her symptoms went away for a short time but came back with a vengeance 2 weeks later. All her X-Rays and blood tests were normal. I sent her to physical therapy. This didn't improve her backache. I started treating her with homeopathy and acupuncture. I started addressing the underlying problems and my 15 minutes office visit turned into a one hour office visit each time she came to see me. With my help, she slowly started appreciating the wonderful things she had, she broke up with her boyfriend and is now happily married to a wonderful man. Her backaches stopped and she hasn't complained of a sore throat since.

Think about how much support you have (read the last page of Chapter 7 again – Chapter on sleep).

Appreciate what you have! A lot of people in Africa are starving. They have no running water, no clothes and no roof to sleep under. You have a lot more than them! Appreciate it! Take the time to smell the roses!

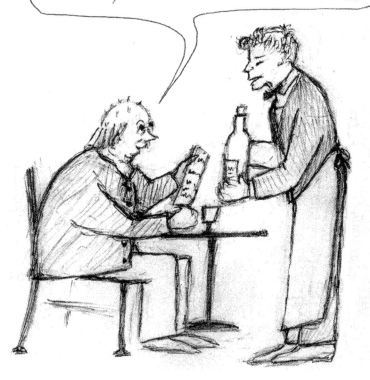

Chapter 15
Take into account your genes

"And remember, no matter where you go, there you are."

Confucius

Your genetic make-up is a critical part of your health and of what you can expect in your lifetime. You already know that the color of your skin, hair and eyes are genetically transmitted from parents to children and sometimes from grand-parents to children, skipping one generation. Well, your susceptibility to diseases is also genetically transmitted. Your genetic make-up will also determine if you will be responsive to a drug or not. It will determine how slowly or fast you will metabolize a drug. Studying this is a new science called pharmacogenetics.

What diseases run in your family? What is your dad suffering from? What is your mom suffering from? What did your grand-parents suffer from? What about your siblings, aunts and uncles?

If one of your parents had angina, a heart attack or a stroke, chances are that you are at higher risk too. This means that diet and exercise are extremely important. Eat salads, fruits, fish and vegetables and make sure you don't get overweight. Exercise one hour per day 5 days a week. Make sure your blood pressure, blood sugar and cholesterol are under control. Make sure you keep your good protective cholesterol in the high norms.

If you are a woman and your mother had breast cancer, you are at higher risk too. Get a genetic screening for BRCA1 (Breast Cancer 1) and BRCA2 gene mutations. If every woman in your family got either breast cancer or ovarian cancer at a young age and if you yourself are carrying the same gene, it is worth getting a bilateral mastectomy with reconstruction and getting both ovaries removed (until we discover better treatments). If there is no breast cancer in your family, make sure you examine your breasts once a month and get a mammogram every year or other year after age 50. If there is any doubt, get an ultrasound and a breast MRI.

If you are a young couple desiring a child, make sure you don't carry the gene mutation responsible for cystic fibrosis. This gene mutation is one of the most 25 common gene mutations in Northern America and there are a lot of normal carriers of this recessive gene. It will give no problem unless a carrier marries another carrier. Then their child has most chances to have cystic fibrosis which is the most common lethal disease in children. Routine carrier screening (can be done by scraping the sides of the mouth) has to be offered legally to every couple who want to conceive or who are already pregnant. It is called predictive genetics.

We now know the gene mutations responsible for familial Alzheimer's disease, colon cancer and many others like factor V Linden mutation. The factor V Linden mutation is a common one and people won't know they carry it until they get a blood clot in their leg after a long flight for example. Those people need to be on anticoagulant therapy because they are at risk of blood clots and sudden death..

If one of your direct parents had colon cancer before the age of 60, you are at higher risk too. Make sure you get regular colonoscopies starting at 50 years old or at least 10 years before the age at which it was first diagnosed in your parent.

If there is diabetes in your family, decrease your sugar intake. If your fasting blood sugar is slightly elevated or your triglycerides are elevated, you need close medical follow-up. Eat as little processed food as possible! Most processed food contains sugar one way or another. Diabetics should eat 5 small meals per day (one small meal every 2 to 3 hours) and avoid high glycemic index foods (See Chapter 4 – foods for diabetic patients).

If you have fair skin and have difficulty getting a tan, you are at higher risk of skin cancer. The fairest your skin is, the most at risk of skin cancer you are if your skin is exposed to the sun for long hours. Those skin cancers can be basal cell carcinoma, squamous cell carcinoma and melanoma. Basal cell and squamous cell skin cancers usually develop on sun exposed areas of the body such as the face, ears, neck and the back of the hands. Basal cell skin cancers are slow growing and rarely metastasize. Melanomas on the other hand are much more aggressive, can arise anywhere in the body and their metastasis can be deadly (brain metastasis).

My patient, E. used to sunbathe a lot when she was younger. She never used sunscreen. Her skin had difficulty getting a tan. She stopped sunbathing when she turned 35 years old and remained healthy for a long time. Suddenly when she turned 50, she noticed a small pearly red lesion on her chest. She went to see her dermatologist who diagnosed a basal cell carcinoma (skin cancer). Now, even though she stopped sunbathing, the damage to her skin is done and she might get new skin cancers every 2 or 3 years.

Use sunscreen cream on every inch of exposed skin with at least SPF 15 and make sure it protects against UVAs and UVBs. If you have a very fair skin, spend a lot of time at the beach with your friends and try to get a nice tan because it is the "in" thing to do, you might have a very high price to pay for this later in your life.

When I was doing my residency, I was called one day by the E.R. to examine B. She was a strikingly beautiful 35 year old woman accompanied by her fiancee. She was in great physical shape since she was a body builder. B. and her fiancee were planning on getting married the following month. She was complaining of weakness in her left hand and arm. This had started one week prior, had gotten slightly better for a few days and was now getting worse. I examined her and found no other significant element than a very slight muscular weakness in her left hand. I sent her for a brain MRI and to my surprise saw a mass in her right brain about 3 centimeters diameter. I showed the mass to the radiologist who pointed out to me one smaller mass about 1.5 centimeters diameter in another area of her brain. Together, we started looking closely at the whole MRI and found 9 other masses ranging from 0.5 to 1cm diameter. She had a total of 11 brain tumors. I was in shock. According to the radiologist, the most likely diagnosis with such an MRI on a young woman was brain metastasis of melanoma. I went back to my patient and asked her about her previous sun exposures. She said she used to lie down in the sun for hours in order to get a nice tan. She was still doing it from time to time but not as much as she used to. I told her what the MRI had shown. She started crying.

Shortly after, we scheduled her for a brain tumor biopsy which showed metastatic melanoma. I looked at her skin but couldn't find any lesion on her skin at all. I learned that skin cancers triggered by sun exposure can appear and disappear spontaneously. When they disappear, they can metastasize. Their favorite spot to metastasize to is the brain.

With 11 tumors in her brain, the prognosis was poor. We offered her to start chemotherapy and radiation therapy explaining to her that it was probably only palliative and would not cure her. We didn't know any treatment to cure her. She decided not to do anything. Later I learned that she got married as scheduled and went on a wonderful honeymoon. She died 6 months later.

So, listen to my advice: wear a hat, long sleeves shirt and pants when you are outside between 10:00 am and 3:00 pm. Use sunscreen creams on all exposed skin.

If you think that one very thin and short layer of sexy clothing with no sleeves and a deep V neck will protect you, think again! You not only need one layer of thin clothing, you need 2 layers to protect you against UVAs and Bs. A dark colored piece of clothing will protect you more that a light one. But if it becomes wet from sweat for example, it will protect you less.

On the bright side, some families live in their 90's and 100's. They have a "longevity" gene and are much less susceptible to diseases. If you are from one of those families, you are very lucky. Chances are you will also live in your 90's or 100's. Most of us unfortunately don't have that gene.

Genetic testing is a new wonderful tool. You can now get genetically tested to find what diseases you are susceptible to. This will probably be used more and more in the future. It will allow you to prevent the diseases you are at risk of developing and if you get them, pharmacogenetics will allow physicians to find the right treatment for you.

Chapter 16
If a medical problem arises, act quickly!

"One does what one is; one becomes what one does."

Robert Von Musil – Kleine prosa

What you do at the very beginning of a medical problem is usually critical.

I'll take a very simple example: Let's say you banged your thigh very violently against a table. You have 10 seconds to act. If you immediately press firmly on the area with your hand and apply pressure for 3 minutes, the bruising, bleeding and swelling will be substantially minimized. After 3 minutes, you can decide whether to apply ice or a cold pack for 10 minutes and then later a cream like Arnica cream. If you don't apply pressure within the first 10 seconds, your vessels will vasoconstrict first in reaction to shock and then, after 10 to 20 seconds, they will be a massive vasodilatation, your small vessels are at a high rupture risk and you might have a huge hematoma which could be very painful and take time to resolve. What you do in the first 10 seconds is very important.

Let's take another example: If you are suddenly experiencing intense chest pain at rest in the early morning as if an elephant is standing on your chest preventing you to breathe, you need to call 911 and be transported to a hospital urgently. While you are waiting for the paramedics to arrive, take one aspirin. Chest pain can be a symptom of a massive heart attack and the prognosis is far better if it is treated right away. One hour can make a huge difference. Within one hour at the hospital, your doctor can diagnose a major blockage in a main artery that brings blood to the heart and treat it which could save your heart from the irreparable damage that could be caused by a delay in treatment.

Now to more complex cases:

If you are suddenly experiencing difficulty speaking or moving one hand or leg, call 911 right away and arrange to be transported to a major hospital urgently. Your diagnosis could be an acute stroke and your treatment will be best if it's administered in the first 2 hours and no later than 3 hours after the onset of your symptoms. A stroke could be caused by a blood clot in one of the main arteries of your brain. You could get immense benefit from a clot retriever device or an intra-venous infusion of a clot dissolver substance. Unfortunately, most hospitals won't use those if it has been more than 3 hours since the onset of your symptoms.

If you are experiencing the worse headache of your life and are vomiting at the same time, arrange to be transported to a major hospital right away. There could be a vessel bleeding in your brain. Treating it right away could save your life.

If you are a woman and find a small lump in your breast, you need to see a doctor as soon as possible. Forget about waiting a few weeks to see if it disappears. One of my patients did just that and she came to see me 9 months after finding a small lump in her breast. By that time her lump was 2 and a half inches diameter and it was too late to treat her breast cancer. She died 6 months later. Had she come to see me within a week of finding her lump, she could have been cured by now.

A lot of cancers have a much better prognosis when they are diagnosed and treated early.

I have a personal example of my own father who died of colon cancer. Had he done regular colonoscopies, his cancer could have been removed at an early stage and he might still be alive now. His first colonoscopy was done 3 months after he found blood in his stools almost every day. His cancer, when it was discovered was too advanced to be cured completely. If you find blood in your stools or in your urine, don't wait and consult your doctor as soon as possible.

Better be safe than sorry. Consult your physician at the beginning of any new symptom.

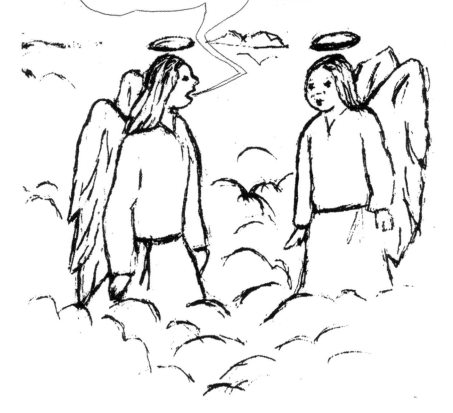

Chapter 17
Don't hesitate to get a second
or even a third opinion

"An in the end, it's not the years in your life that count,
it's the life in your years."

Abraham Lincoln

For major health problems, it can be important to have the opinion of 2 or 3 specialist physicians. Most of the time, the treatments will be the same but sometimes you will be very surprised to see that they can differ tremendously. In which case, you need to choose the treatment that is most appropriate for you and makes the most sense. You might need the help of your family doctor to determine which specialist to trust the most.

Even the best physician can make medical mistakes. A physician sees an average of 20 to 40 patients a day, usually a different patient every 15 minutes. This makes an average of 100 to 200 patients a week. Even with the best training, experience and intention, it is inevitable that medical mistakes happen. By getting a 2nd and sometimes a 3rd opinion, you will reduce this chance of mistake.

When my Dad was diagnosed with liver metastasis from his colon cancer, he went to see his gastro-enterologist who recommended extremely painful alcohol injections directly in the tumor itself. Dad, trusting his physician did exactly what he recommended. When I came back from Mauritania where I was working for Doctors Without Borders, I accompanied him to his doctors' office. I witnessed the extremely painful alcohol injection in the liver tumor. Dad was screaming with pain on the procedure table. Since the injection was guided by an ultrasound, I asked the physician what the diameter of the tumor was. I was horrified to hear that despite the injections, the tumor was still growing fast. I convinced Dad to stop his injections and I went to present his case to all the best cancer specialists in all the major hospitals in Paris. I was surprised to hear that each and every one of them had a different opinion. One of them said chemotherapy was the best way to go. It wouldn't cure him but it could postpone his death. Another one recommended that we do nothing and just let him die peacefully. A third one told me about a new procedure that could potentially save him. He would cut his abdomen open, remove half of his liver and have him receive chemotherapy afterwards. All of them had one opinion in common: Alcohol injections had not been useful in any patient with liver metastasis anywhere in the world. The last physician made the most sense to me. Dad was still strong enough to go through a difficult surgery. Surgically removing half of his liver (the half that contained the metastasis which was now 7 centimeter – almost 3 inches - diameter) was the way to go. This surgery was successful and gave him several more years of life. The most surprising thing was to see how fast his liver grew back to its normal size after the surgery. Within 2 months after the surgery, his liver had a normal size again and Dad was completely tumor-free.

If you are experiencing symptoms that don't require urgent treatment and you are not sure you want to follow the recommendations of the doctor you just saw, get a second or even a third opinion from reputable specialist physicians. You will then make your final decision of what to do taking into account your goal, your age, the insurance coverage you have and your own financial resources.

Chapter 18
When to use Alternative Medicine

"Believe those who are seeking the truth. Doubt those who find it."

Andre Gide

Conventional Medicine, Alternative Medicine, Homeopathy, Acupuncture and Herbs are all wonderful when they are used appropriately. The key word here is appropriately.

For the beginning of a cold or the first day of diarrhea, use alternative medicine first. Most of the time, your symptoms will go away within 48 hours. If they don't, you might need conventional medications.

On the other hand, do not use Alternative Medicine as a main therapy to fight against cancer. For cancer, always use Conventional Therapy as a main therapy. In addition and only in addition, you can use Alternative Medicines to help you fight against the side effects of chemotherapy and for anti-cancer action.

Do not use Alternative Medicine as a main therapy to fight against a heart attack. After a heart attack, always use Conventional Therapy as a main therapy also and then add Alternative Medicine to finish the job.

Now, let's talk about chronic fatigue syndrome: If all your test results are normal, always use Homeopathy and/ or Acupuncture first. With

Homeopathy and Acupuncture, you will have no side effect and no drug interaction. If they work, you will be cured. If they don't, then, it will be time to go to Conventional Medicine.

For any new symptom, first consult your primary care physician to make a diagnosis and start an urgent treatment if needed. Your physician will determine whether you can use alternative medicine, homeopathy, acupuncture or herbs or if you absolutely need conventional medications.

For this, make sure your physician spends enough time with you to comprehend your problem. I usually spend at least one hour face to face with a patient on the first office visit if the case is complex. It takes me at least one hour to carefully listen to each complaint, ask questions, examine my patient, explain the treatment I suggest and document our encounter. Very few physicians will spend an hour face to face with you which is O.K. as long as they understand what your problem is.

Ideally, the first office visit should be an extensive one, making sure that you are eating the right way, drinking the right beverages, exercising enough, sleeping enough, spending quality time with yourself and with your mate, spending time with family and friends and finding time for your hobby and passion in life. I try to make sure you are spinning all those plates at the right speed for you. I need to review not only all the medications you take but also all the over-the-counter supplements you take. Some supplements in contrast with pure homeopathic medicines, have side effects and drug interactions. I need to make sure you are not taking too high doses of those supplements but also that you are taking enough of the right supplement for you. I need to carefully examine you and then explain you your diagnosis and the different possible ways to treat you. All this takes time and is key for a successful treatment and a satisfied patient. Medicine cannot be the same for everybody. It needs to be tailored to each patient.

Make sure you choose the right physician for you.

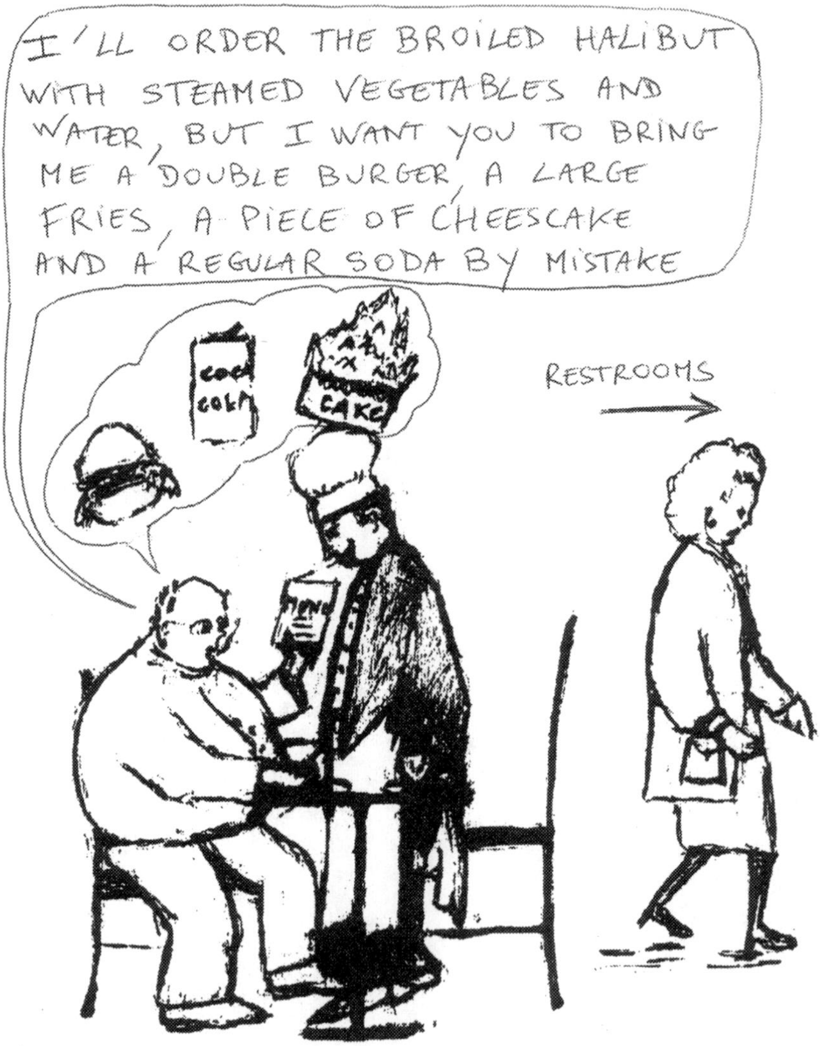
I'LL ORDER THE BROILED HALIBUT WITH STEAMED VEGETABLES AND WATER, BUT I WANT YOU TO BRING ME A DOUBLE BURGER, A LARGE FRIES, A PIECE OF CHEESCAKE AND A REGULAR SODA BY MISTAKE
CAKE
RESTROOMS

Chapter 19
Vitamins and Nutritional Supplements

*"He who takes medicines and neglects to diet wastes the skill
of his doctors."*

Chinese proverb

A little tablet of <u>multivitamin</u> every day will give you all the vitamins
your body needs.

If you don't eat milk products and are not outside in the sun 15
minutes a day, make sure you take at least 1000 to 1200 mg of <u>Calcium</u>
(Calcium Citrate is absorbed the best by the guts) and 800 to 1,000
international units of <u>Vitamin D</u> per day to prevent osteoporosis.

We are now finding that a lot of patients are <u>Vitamin D</u> deficient.
Vitamin D is in reality a hormone. It is made by the skin after sun
exposure. 15 minutes per day in the sun with shorts and short sleeves
shirt between 10:00 am and 3:00 pm will give you all the Vitamin
D you need. If you stay longer in the sun, you will be at risk of skin
cancer. Sunscreen cream more than 8 SPF, clothing, glass and plastic
windows will impair the photosynthesis of Vitamin D. Some foods
also contain Vitamin D: one tablespoon of Cod liver oil will bring
you 1,360 international units of Vitamin D, 3 oz of Salmon with bring
you 794 units, 3 oz of Mackerel: 388 units, one cup of fortified milk:

120 units, 6 oz of Yoghurt: 80 units. Research is currently done on the benefits of Vitamin D which seem to be boosting the immune system, strengthening bone formation, endocrine system and vessels walls. Recently published articles show that it could reduce aggressiveness of cancers, reduce expansion of atheromatous lesions, severity of type 2 diabetes and could decrease all cause mortality. Ask your doctor to measure the Vitamin D level in your blood.

Since Calcium tends to make people constipated and Magnesium tends to give diarrhea, a lot of manufacturers are now adding Magnesium to Calcium in the same tablet.

Your body needs some good fats in the form of Omega-3 fatty acids - EPA (Eicosapentaenoic acid), DHA (Docosahexaenoic acid) and ALA (Alpha linolenic acid) -which are found in Flax seed oil, perilla seed oil, fish oil, and CLA (conjugated linoleic acid). Those are wonderful for the heart, blood vessels in general and for the brain.

If you have joint pains, Glucosamine-Chondroitin (at least 1200 mg per day) has shown in some studies to improve joint health.

If you have inflammatory or irritable bowel syndrome or if you are on antibiotics, Probiotics (Acidophilus) with at least 4 billion organisms twice a day has shown to significantly decrease bowel inflammation.

For liver problems, milk thistle is the supplement you want to take since it seems to improve liver health.

For enlarged prostate, Saw Palmetto 320 mg per day has shown in some studies it could improve prostate health.

For hot flashes due to menopause, black cohosh has shown great improvements in some studies.

Macular degeneration is one of the causes of gradual loss of vision which can lead to blindness. To slow it down, the combination 500 mg of vitamin C + 400 International Units of Vitamin E + 15 mg beta carotene + 80 mg Zinc oxide + 2 mg of copper as cupric oxide orally per day has shown to be effective in some studies.

To prevent cancer, some specialists recommend <u>selenium</u> 100 to 200 mcg per day. Selenium is contained in brazil nuts: 2 brazil nuts per day will bring the perfect dose of Selenium you need.

<u>Chromium Picolinate</u> could help diabetes by helping metabolize glucose.

<u>Garlic</u> and <u>Ginkgo biloba</u> will make your blood thinner which could prevent strokes. Garlic could also work as an antiviral and antibacterial.

<u>Folic acid</u>, <u>Vitamin B6</u> and <u>B12</u> could make your heart stronger.

<u>Coenzyme Q 10</u> could help all the metabolisms in your body and could make you feel less tired.

<u>Cranberry juice</u> could help you fight against urinary tract infections (E. Coli) and stomach infections (H. Pylori).

But be careful since too high doses of some vitamins can cause damage. Too high a dose of vitamin A could increase your risk of bone fracture. Too high a dose of vitamin E could be cardio toxic.

Be very careful with over-the-counter nutritional supplements and always tell your doctor about the supplements you are taking. Some supplements can have terrible side effects and can interact with conventional medications making them either inactive or too active even toxic.

For example:

<u>Ephedra</u> can cause high blood pressure, irregular heart beat, strokes and even heart attacks. Sometimes instead of using its name Ephedra,

people use its other names: Epitonin, Ma huang, Mahuuanggen, Muzei mu huang, Natural Ecstasy, Pinellia, Popotillo, Sea grape, Sida cordifolia, Yellow horse, Zhong ma huang, Bitter Orange or Citrus Aurantium. Look at all the ingredients of all the supplements you buy. If one of the ingredients is listed above, do not buy it. It could be really toxic.

St. John's wort indicated for mild depression interacts with conventional medications. It reduces the efficacy of other medicine like birth control pills, SSRIs (a type of antidepressant), theophylline, antiepileptics, pravastatin, digoxin, warfarin, loperamide, cyclosporine, chemotherapy drugs and anti HIV drugs. If you are a woman on birth control pills, by taking St John's wort you might get less depressed but you might also get pregnant...

One week before surgery, stop echinacea, fish oil, garlic, ginger, ginkgo, ginseng, kava, St John's wort, valerian and vitamin E which can interfere with anesthesia or can make you bleed more.

As more and more people take supplements, more and more side effects and drug interactions are being discovered. Supplements are not FDA controlled and regulated. If they are not regulated in the United States, they are even less regulated elsewhere which means that they can contain anything and everything. Some of them do not contain what the label says they contain. Instead of containing 25 mg of active product (which is written on the label), they may only contain 1 mg or sometimes 0 mg. Others are not pure. They may contain contaminants like lead, arsenic or anabolic hormones which are toxic. Some people have had acute liver failure needing liver transplant after taking contaminated supplements.

M. came to see me complaining of diarrhea for 3 months. I reviewed all the medications and supplements she was taking and discovered that she was taking 10 different supplements. Each of the supplement contained several ingredients: Magnesium was in 5 of those. I calculated the amount of Magnesium she was taking per day. It was over 1500 mg per day. This was the origin of her diarrhea. As soon as she changed supplements and decreased her intake of Magnesium, her diarrhea stopped.

Part of the office visit with your doctor should be to discuss all the supplements you are taking in order to review their necessity. Some people come to me with a whole suitcase of nutritional supplements they are taking every day. This is usually too much. Unless your guts don't absorb the food you are eating, chances are that if you eat a balanced diet with fruits, salads and vegetables every day you don't need most of the supplements and vitamins you are taking. As a matter of fact, some studies are starting to show that instead of making you live longer, taking a lot of vitamins and supplements could make you die sooner.

Make sure you can discuss this topic with your physician.

Chapter 20
Hormones

"From the bitterness of disease, man learns the sweetness of health"

Catalan proverb

When you don't feel good, feel fatigued, have intense hot flashes, gain or lose weight, it is worth getting your hormones checked. The basic serum hormonal panel I like to prescribe is:

For thyroid function: Free T3 (thyroid hormone), free T4 (thyroid hormone), TSH (pituitary gland hormone).

For Adrenal gland function: Cortisol.

For women: DHEA-Sulfate (hormone precursor), Estradiol, Progesterone, FSH (pituitary gland hormone), Total Testosterone, Sex hormone binding Globulin (protein making sex hormones inactive).

For men: DHEA-Sulfate (hormone precursor), Total Testosterone, Sex Hormone Binding Globulin (protein making Testosterone inactive).

Knowing the level of Sex Hormone Binding Globulin allows me to calculate the amount of free therefore active hormones. For example, some people can have a normal level of Total Testosterone but have a very high level of Sex Hormone Binding Globulin which will bind most of their Testosterone making most of it inactive. The calculated level of Free Testosterone becomes therefore too low. They feel fatigued and have a very low sex drive. Those people need Testosterone replacement therapy.

Emerging data show that men who have a very low Testosterone level have more cardiovascular disease and more severe prostate cancer. The lower their Testosterone is the more visceral obesity they tend to have. They also have high triglycerides, high cholesterol, insulin resistance, low bone mineral density and low sex drive. Surprisingly enough, recent studies show that if they have prostate cancer, the lower their Testosterone is at baseline, the worse their prognosis is. Unfortunately there are no safety data yet to support long term Testosterone replacement therapy. We still need adequate randomized trials.

P. was a 45 year old man who came to see me 2 years ago because he was tired all the time, had a very low sex drive and was overweight. I measured his morning Total Testosterone level which was 230 which was pretty low. His Sex Hormone Binding Globulin was high which made most of his Testosterone inactive. I started him on Testosterone in form of a gel to apply on his skin every morning. Within one month, he was feeling spectacularly better. Within 3 months, he was feeling as energetic as when he was 30 years old, his sex drive came back which made him and his wife very happy, his memory improved and he became much more efficient at his job. He started losing weight, having more lean muscle mass and strength, stronger bones and started exercising regularly. He is still applying his Testosterone gel on his skin every morning. I check his prostate and blood test twice a year. He says "life is wonderful again!"

B. was a 52 year old lady who came to see me because she was having terrible hot flashes ever since she stopped having her periods 2 years ago. Her physician didn't give her any hormone replacement therapy because of the risk of breast cancer. B. felt really miserable and her quality of life was very poor. At night, she was woken up every hour and a half by profuse sweating. She was drenched. Indeed, when she was touching her skin, it was as wet as if she had just gotten out of the shower! Her sheets were soaked! She had to change sheets at least 3 times per night. It was a horrible experience! During the day, she felt very tired and 10 to 11 times a day, her face would become bright red and suddenly, she would start sweating profusely for a few seconds to a few minutes. It was very embarrassing since it always happened when she was in meetings. She had to take off her sweater and then after a few minutes would become cold and had to put her sweater on again. She had a very low quality of life and needed help. I tested her hormones and found a very low level of Estradiol, Progesterone, Total Testosterone and DHEA-Sulfate. She clearly needed hormonal supplementation. The treatment with bio-identical Estradiol cream, Natural Progesterone, Testosterone and DHEA changed her life. Her hot flashes stopped; she started sleeping again; her fatigue resolved; her libido which had completely disappeared came back which made her husband really happy.

B. was aware that hormone replacement therapy even with bio-identical hormones had pros and cons:

List of possible complications due to hormone replacement therapy:-

- It increases the risk of blood clots, coronary events, heart attacks, strokes, pulmonary embolisms, deep venous thrombosis,
- It increases the risk of breast cancer
- It increases the risk of endometrial uterine cancer
- increases the risk of liver and gallbladder problems,
- increases the risk of weight gain,
- increases triglycerides,
- if estrogens and progesterone are taken without Testosterone, they can decrease libido by decreasing the level of Free Testosterone

On the other hand, the benefits of Hormone Replacement Therapy are:

- Suppress hot flashes,
- Decrease the risk of colon cancer,
- Increase the good HDL cholesterol,
- They help fight against osteoporosis and bone fracture,
- Good for the skin (anti-aging)

In B's case, the suppression of hot flashes made such a difference in her life that she was ready to accept the risks. We chose the lowest possible dose of hormones which also lowered her risks and she started appreciating every single minute of her life again.

S. was another very nice lady who was complaining of weakness, fatigue, constipation, dry skin and depression. She was cold all the time and had started gaining weight in the last few months. Her hair was thinning and her nails were becoming brittle. She had headaches and muscle cramps.

Her blood test showed that her thyroid gland was not functioning well any more. She needed thyroid hormone therapy which I gave her in the form of combination of Triiodothyronine (T3) and Thyroxine (T4). Within a few months she lost all the weight she had gained and her symptoms disappeared.

You too might need your hormones checked and depending on the results, might need hormone replacement therapy. You may want to ask your physician for a basic hormonal panel.

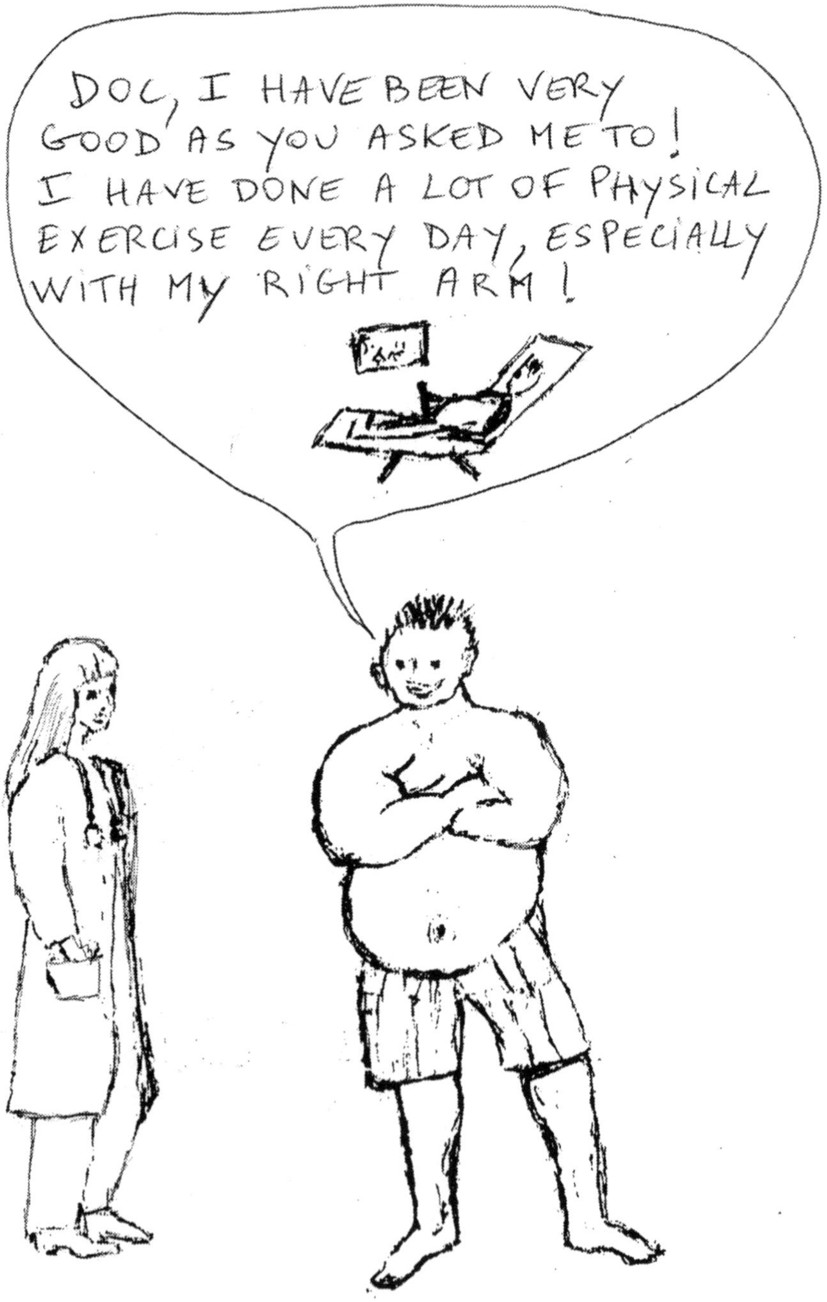
DOC, I HAVE BEEN VERY GOOD AS YOU ASKED ME TO! I HAVE DONE A LOT OF PHYSICAL EXERCISE EVERY DAY, ESPECIALLY WITH MY RIGHT ARM!

Chapter 21
Homeopathy and Acupuncture

"The obstacle is the path."

Zen proverb

Conventional medications can be very effective but equally aggressive and have sometimes a lot of potentially dangerous side effects. For cases when conventional medications are not absolutely needed, people who often have better results with homeopathy or acupuncture.

Acupuncture is based on the principle that there are energetic pathways called meridians throughout the body that influence how internal organs function. It is used in traditional Chinese Medicine and has been practiced for at least 2500 years. In my office, I usually rebalance my patients' 12 major meridians using extremely fine gauge needles or electrical stimulation at key acupuncture points. It allows their Qi or vital force to flow more freely and keeps their forces of Yin and Yang in balance.

Homeopathy uses highly diluted doses of herbs, minerals and animal extracts. The theory behind homeopathy is that "like cures like": A very diluted dose of a particular plant, mineral or animal extract treats symptoms that could be generated by the same extract if given in toxic doses. For example a large dose of onion will give us runny nose and watery eyes. If we come down with a cold with runny nose and watery eyes, we can benefit from <u>Allium Cepa</u> 12 C (Allium Cepa means onion in Latin) which is made with onion extract diluted 12 times one hundred times. It usually works very well. It's a different way of treating, gentle and safe. If homeopathy doesn't work, then it is time for conventional medication.

When I talk about homeopathy, I generally talk about medicines that have a C after their names which means they are diluted at least one hundred times. Some people call homeopathy medicines diluted ten times only or even mother tinctures which are the pure extract of the plant. In the USA, mother tinctures are also called 1X. They are the pure extract used to prepare the different dilutions and they are as close to conventional medicine as you can get. Those 1X preparations have side effects and drug interactions like any conventional medicine. Make sure you look at all the ingredients of all the over-the-counter medications you are buying.

Homeopathy with C (centesimal) dilutions is wonderful for children. Here is an example:

B. 5 years old had been on antibiotics once or twice a month for the last 6 months. She had alternating otitis (ear infections), pharyngitis (throat infections) and bronchitis. When her mother brought her to me, 2 years ago, she was just starting to have a sore throat again. B. was a very pretty little girl, slim and very active. Her throat was bright red. She had no fever and wanted to have cold drinks to relieve her sore throat. I gave her <u>Apis Mellifica</u> 12 C (12 C dilutions are diluted 12 times one hundred times) 5 pellets 3 times a day and within a couple of days, her sore throat resolved without antibiotics. I looked for her personal constitutional homeopathic remedy which I determined was <u>Calcarea Phosphorica</u>. I gave her Calcarea Phosphorica 12 C 5 pellets every morning when waking up. In the last couple of years, I only gave her antibiotics once. She has been feeling much better and stronger with Homeopathy. I told her Mom to address each of B's symptoms right away with the appropriate homeopathic treatment as soon as they start:

Here is a list of very useful medications that I told her to use either in 12 C or 30C:

Aconitum Napellus for any symptom happening suddenly after cold and dry weather. To be given when B's skin is warm and dry and when B is agitated and thirsty.

Dulcamara for any symptom happening after a rain or a bath (notion of being exposed to water or humidity in general).

Apis Mellifica for fever with warm skin and lack of thirst. All symptoms are improved by cold applications. Everything is worse with heat and with touch.

Belladona for fever with intense thirst. The patient is hypersensitive to light, touch and noise, tends to be agitated; the skin is red and there is sweating particularly from the face. The main difference between Aconitum Napellus and Belladona is that Aconitum Napellus should be given if there is no sweating and Belladona if there is sweating.

Bryonia Alba for fever with headache, muscle pain or joint pain that are worse with movement; dry cough also worse with movement. Everything is better when the patient doesn't move. He or she has to stay still or lie still in bed to feel better. There is sweating and intense thirst that can leave a bitter taste in the mouth.

Drosera Rotundifolia for spasmodic dry cough worse at night after midnight when lying in a warm bed, worse when speaking and singing.

Ferrum Phosphoricum for a fever that is not very high. The skin is moist. The face is pale at times and flushed at other times. There is often ear pain and there can be bleeding from the nose.

<u>Kali Bichromicum</u> for productive cough or sinus infection with thick yellow greenish secretions worse with cold weather and between 2 and 3 am.

<u>Kali Iodatum</u> for watery eyes, sneezing, profuse watery discharge from the nose which is red, swollen and very painful.

<u>Kali Muriaticum</u> for middle ear and tonsil inflammation worse with cold damp air.

<u>Phytolacca Decandra</u> for sore throat worse in cold and damp weather.

Using Homeopathy on children at the first symptom allows the treatment to work very quickly without side effect or drug interaction. Homeopathy works wonderfully most of the time. The one time it didn't work on B., I prescribed antibiotics but this was only once in 2 years which is much better than once or twice a month.

Homeopathic medicines taste good and children love them. They are also very cheap and readily available in most health food stores without a prescription.

Here is another example:

V. was a 51 year old pleasant lady who came to see me 8 months ago for the first time, referred by her best friend. She had been feeling depressed for the last 4 weeks. Her depression started when her Mom passed away from cancer. V. took care of her Mom the last 6 months of her life. V. felt that she had given her Mom every drop of energy she had. She was now completely exhausted, had frequent headaches and was hypersensitive to noise.

I started by giving her <u>Arnica Montana</u> 30 C 10 pellets under the tongue once to address the origin of her depression. Arnica Montana is the mountain daisy. It is wonderful after a shock. It can be a physical shock like a fall in which case I like to give it in 6 C dilution (diluted 6 times one hundred times). It is also wonderful after an emotional shock in which case I give it in 30 C dilution (diluted 30 times one hundred times). I also prescribed <u>Phosphoricum Acidum</u> 30 C 5 pellets under the tongue 3 times a day. Phosphoricum Acidum (Phosphoric Acid) works wonders for grief in the context of physical and mental exhaustion. At the same time I did Acupuncture on her, using in particular the Heart 3 point at the elbow which is a wonderful anti-depression point. I saw V. once a week for the next 3 weeks. Each week, she got progressively better. After 3 weeks, she was almost back to normal. Had she not improved, I would have prescribed a conventional anti-depression treatment but conventional medicines can have side effects which I wasn't ready to risk yet. With Arnica Montana and Phosphoricum Acidum, there was no side effect, no drug interaction, the treatment worked quickly and was very cheap.

The following month, V. told her husband to come and see me. F. was a very busy 56 year old executive in a large firm. He was complaining of being fatigued and bloated all the time. He had a lot of gas which made his abdomen very sensitive day and night. He was very sedentary, working long hours at his computer without moving and was not exercising at all. He was eating too much and was grossly overweight. I gave him <u>Nux Vomica</u> 12 C 5 pellets under the tongue 3 times a day, to be taken 10 to 15 minutes before meals. I used Acupuncture with mostly the Large Intestine 4 on his hands and I told him to change his life style. He had to start physical exercise with a 30 minutes walk every morning. He had to get up from his desk at least every hour to stretch and walk. He had to eat lighter meals. Within a few months, F. improved tremendously. He lost 20 lbs, had no more bloating and was feeling much more energetic.

<u>Homeopathy can be used in combination with specific massages for restless leg syndrome, constipation and hypothyroidism.</u>

<u>For restless leg syndrome</u>, Zincum Metallicum 6 C or 12 C works wonders in combination with the following leg massage: lie down, put your legs up against a wall or the head of your bed, apply <u>Arnica gel</u> on your legs massaging them from your ankles to your thighs.

The movement should be free flowing bringing blood from your legs towards your heart. Massage with Arnica gel and sucking on Zincum Metallicum pellets should be done at bedtime and also as needed during the day.

For constipation, Alumina 12 C 5 pellets every morning when getting up works well. At the same time, massage your belly 3 times every morning. The belly massage is very precise: lie down, put your right hand on top of your nightgown, pyjama or a tee shirt on the lower right part of your belly then with a very light pressure bring your hand towards the upper right part of your belly close to your ribs, move it slowly towards the upper left part then towards the lower left part. Lift your hand up and start again at the lower right part. Do this 3 to 5 times in a row before getting up. The pressure you need to apply shouldn't be too hard and it shouldn't hurt.

For mild hypothyroidism (when the thyroid gland doesn't work enough), Thyroidinum 6 X 5 pellets under the tongue every morning has been consistently very helpful to a lot of patients. At the same time, massage the Stomach 9 acupuncture point 10 times every morning. The Stomach 9 acupuncture point is located on both side of the throat, very close to the thyroid gland itself.

Homeopathy and Acupuncture can also be used with Conventional Medicine. Here is one case:

M. was a 59 year old woman who was on chemotherapy for ovarian cancer. She absolutely needed her regular doses of chemo to keep the cancer at bay. Unfortunately, her chemo was giving her a lot of side effects. I used Homeopathy and Acupuncture to address those side effects. Ipecacuanha 12 C 5 pellets under the tongue 3 times a day worked wonderfully to decrease her nausea. Podophyllum Peltatum worked on her diarrhea which was watery and worse in the early morning. As for acupuncture, I gave her a session every week for 4 weeks then once a month, rebalancing her meridians and using anti-nausea and anti-diarrhea points. The result was spectacular.

At the beginning of this book, I talked about chronic fatigue syndrome. I see more and more people coming to me with this diagnosis. They usually need a whole work-up done by their internist to rule out major causes like hormonal problems, infection or cancer. Once everything is ruled out, since the internist has no treatment to offer, the patient is referred to me. In order to treat the patient adequately, I always need to know how things started. What triggered the beginning of the symptoms? It could be a shock in which case I give Arnica Montana. It could be an infection with a E. Coli bacteria in which case I give Colibacillinum in a high dilution. It could be a Staphylococcus infection in which case I give Staphylococcinum in a high dilution. Whatever the trigger is, I address it by giving the appropriately targeted homeopathic treatment.

Then, I concentrate on the progression of symptoms that my patient had and on the details about the current symptoms. I determine which toxicology the symptoms are similar to.

One of my patient, D. was complaining of being tired and sick all the time. Everything started when she was 32 years old and had a very severe flu. Since then she has been cold all the time, had recurrent bronchitis and urinary tract infections; her nails were brittle and she was sweating profusely especially from the feet; her head was always cold and she frequently needed to wear a hat; she had frequent abscesses and dental infections; she was constipated and was not sleeping well. Her symptoms were very similar to a Silicea intoxication. She needed a high dilution of Silicea to fight against those symptoms. But to start with, I gave her in a high dilution of Influenzinum since everything started after a severe flu, then I gave her Silicea in progressively higher and higher dilutions. I also gave her an acupuncture session once a week. Very quickly she started improving tremendously. After two months, she was almost back to normal.

2 magical little known homeopathic medicines are Venus Mercenaria and Raphanus Sativus Niger.

Venus Mercenaria works wonderfully on headaches. Very few people know about it and I have prescribed it to numerous patients with a high success rate. Of course, first we need to make sure that the headache is not due to a tumor, trauma, infection, vascular malformation or any other cause that warrants urgent conventional treatment. Some people have headaches regularly; no explanation can be found and their brain MRI, CT scan and blood tests are all normal; in those cases Venus Mercenaria diluted 30 times one hundred times (30C) can make wonders.

The other little known medicine is Raphanus Sativus Niger (Black Radish) which works great diluted 6 times one hundred times (6C) on constipation with gas retention: S. had had gallbladder surgery 2 days prior. She was feeling very bloated and couldn't pass any gas. I gave her Raphanus Sativus Niger 6 C five pellets under the tongue 4 times a day. Within 8 hours she passed a loud gas and 5 hours later she had a bowel movement.

I do use homeopathy myself. My favorite ones are Oscillococcinum which I take at the first sign of flu or cold and Histaminum since I tend to have hay fever. I also used Gelsemium Sempervirens a lot in my life to get less emotional before an exam. I took Gelsemium Sempervirens 12 C or 30 C 5 pellets the evening before each of my exam and 5 pellets the morning of. With this on board, I got much less emotional (I used to panic at exams) and always got excellent grades. Gelsemium 30 C is made with the plant Yellow Jasmine diluted 30 times 100 times. Again, it has no side effect or drug interaction since it is so diluted.

The wonderful thing about homeopathy is that the medications are readily available at most health food stores without a prescription and they are very affordable.

Chapter 22
Medical secrets and myths

"Courage is what it takes to stand up and speak; courage is also what it takes to sit down and listen."

Winston Churchill

Here are a few secrets that nobody wants you to know:

Secret # 1:

Avoid taking a new drug which has been on the market for less than one year. If the drug is from a new class of drugs that has just been approved by the FDA, it takes at least one year and sometimes several years to discover its new side effects which could be life threatening.

Secret # 2:

Avoid going to a teaching hospital in the United States at the end of June and in July. Those are the first weeks of the new interns and residents. They are just learning surgery (it can be their first time using a scalpel…) or medicine and there are much more medical mistake being done than at the end of the teaching year in April, May or beginning of June.

Secret # 3:

You cannot blindly trust a physician 100%. Some physicians are only in this for the money and not for your best interest. A lot of physicians will rush patients in order to process as many claims as possible. Some surgeons will recommend surgery even if surgery is not needed. Some physicians who just acquired a new piece of equipment like an ultrasound machine will recommend that you have an ultrasound study even if you don't need it. This way they will get more money from you or your insurance.

Secret # 4:

It is very likely that a general surgeon will know very little about cardiology (heart problems), a cardiologist will know very little about ophthalmology (eye problems), an ophthalmologist will know very little about dermatology (skin problems). Each physician specialist is usually very knowledgeable in his or her own field of expertise but usually knows very little about other medical fields.

Secret # 5:

Even the best physician can make the wrong diagnosis or choose the wrong medication. You need to do your own research on your problem. You might need to consult several specialists to get different opinions. For this, you need to keep copies of your blood results, X-Rays, CT scans, MRI results, etc... which can easily be lost in a large office or hospital. Ultimately, you are your own best primary care physician.

Secret # 6:

Medicine changes constantly as we speak and as I write this book. One year, physicians tell you that hormone replacement therapy is good for women starting menopause. The following year, they tell you it is bad and has too many side effects. Every year and sometimes every month, there are new trends and new discoveries based on ongoing research. Make sure you and your physician keep up to date with what is new.

Secret # 7:

If you hurt yourself, fall on your buttock or bang a part of your body against a hard surface, the first thing to do is to press on the area for 3 minutes. You have 10 seconds to do so. During the first 10 seconds, all the vessels in the injured area get into spasms and vasoconstriction then, after 10 seconds, there is a massive vasodilatation. All the vessels explode and bleed out. There could be a lot of swelling. The fastest way to prevent this is to press on the area immediately and firmly with your hand and do so for 3 minutes without releasing the pressure. Then and only then can you apply ice and afterwards Arnica cream or gel. This way, you will have very little bruising and within a couple of days, you won't even be able to see where the point of impact was.

Steve, my husband, used to do a lot of repairs and construction in our house and hurt himself periodically. Each time, I used to nag him: "Press on it for 3 minutes!" He would press on the area immediately and it prevented all bruising. One day, he fell off the ladder in our yard and scraped his left leg and knee. He looked at his leg, afraid to have broken it. Nothing was showing and he had no pain. He forgot to apply pressure and kept on with his work. Ten minutes later, he ran into the house, screaming "Doctor, doctor, is there a doctor in the house?" Completely panicked, he showed me his leg which had a big scrape, was bleeding and was very swollen. "Did you apply pressure for 3 minutes?" I asked. He said that he forgot and suddenly sat down on the kitchen floor, applying pressure on his leg. I asked him to release the pressure so that I could disinfect the area with iodine. He refused, still pressing on the area. Half an hour later, he was still on the kitchen floor pressing on his leg… When I finally convinced him to release the pressure, the swelling had decreased tremendously. I disinfected his wound with iodine and the following day, his leg looked back to normal. From that time on, he never forgot to apply pressure right away after a trauma.

Secret # 8:

Antibacterial soaps are really not needed in your household. A regular soap is as effective if it is well used. Make sure you wash your hands thoroughly several times a day. Make sure you put a lot of regular soap in between every finger and wash for at least 10 seconds before you rinse.

Secret # 9:

The face creams that are the most expensive are not always the best. A cream that smells really good and has a long list of ingredients in it could be really expensive but it could sensitize your skin too much and be too irritating. Some people become allergic to a lot of creams. Their skin becomes red and itchy. The better the cream smells the more chances you have to be allergic to it. The more ingredients a cream has, the more chances you have to be allergic to one of its components. Ideally, choose a cream that has no scent and that only has a few ingredients. For a day cream, make sure it has a SPF (sun protection factor) of at least 15.

Secret # 10:

More and more people are allergic to pollens, pollution, dust mites and certain types of foods. It could be very difficult to find what a particular person is allergic to. Some people require patch testing in a dermatology office. The symptoms can vary from asthma to hay fever to urticaria. With processed foods containing more and more ingredients, it becomes very complex to find the culprit:

M. had been itching for 8 months. We couldn't find what she was allergic to. We thought it was shrimp, seafood, nuts, a new soap or a new cream. She stopped all of the above and she was still itching. That's when we thought about lettuce. She was eating lettuce every day in order to lose weight. As soon as she stopped eating lettuce, her itching stopped. Lettuce contains Lactucin to which some people can be allergic to. It is not as common as nuts or seafood allergy but it does happen.

T., another patient, had been bloated, fatigued and had had lose stools for 6 months. We did some testing and found out she couldn't digest Gluten. I put her on a Gluten-free diet and her symptoms resolved.

Sometimes, it takes the skill of a detective to find what a particular person is allergic to. Here is an interesting case: S. had noticed sometimes, he couldn't get an erection for 2 weeks. Then, his erections would come back to normal, being an erection every day when waking up. Looking closely at what was different in those 2 weeks, he stated that he was putting some pickles in his lunch sandwich every day and eating curry dishes. That didn't happen the other weeks. Ultimately, we determined he was allergic to turmeric. Looking at the ingredients of the pickles he was eating, we saw that they contained turmeric as a preservative. Each time he ate something with turmeric or curry (which by the way are very healthy and can act as natural anti-inflammatory), he couldn't get an erection for 24 hours. He has been staying away from turmeric and has had no problem with erections ever since.

Secret # 11:

If you drink one large bottle (20 oz) of soda per day, you could gain up to 26 lbs per year. Sodas are loaded with sugar which makes people gain weight.

Secret # 12:

Low-fat diets is not recommended any more. When they used to be recommended, people would say: "it is fat-free, it is good for me, I can eat the whole box!" Fat-free foods are often loaded with sugar! We are now recommending low sugar diet with low glycemic index foods and heart-healthy fats like nuts, olive oil, flaxseed and fish.

Secret # 13:

Some unregulated over-the-counter protein supplements have been found to be contaminated with anabolic steroid hormones which could be very damaging for your health.

Secret # 14:

Over-the-counter non-steroidal anti-inflammatory drugs reduce kidney perfusion and can aggravate an acute renal failure. Make sure you don't take too many Ibuprofen, Aspirin or Naproxen tablets for too long. If you take anti-inflammatory drugs, make sure you drink a lot of water to protect your kidneys.

Secret # 15:

Acetaminophen which is contained in Tylenol can be liver toxic. Make sure you don't take too high doses for too long.

Secret # 16:

After a CT scan or MRI with contrast dye, make sure you drink a lot of water to eliminate the dye properly otherwise it could be kidney toxic.

Here are a few myths:

Myth # 1:

Frogs and toads cause warts. This is a myth. They do not cause warts. Warts are caused by little skin viruses and a very easy and cheap way to get rid of them is to use duct tape. Place a duct tape on your wart, leave it for 6 days, then take it off, soak the area in water, rub the wart with a purnice stone or emery board, leave out for the night then place another duct tape on it, leave it for 6 days, then take it off, soak the area in water, then rub the wart again with a purnice stone or emery board, leave out for the night then do the same procedure again in the morning and again for one to 2 months. After one or 2 months, your wart will have disappeared.

Myth # 2:

Masturbation causes blindness. This is a myth. Masturbation is actually quite healthy. It helps release sexual tension.

Myth # 3:

Dead poison oak plants cannot give a rash. This is a myth. What causes a rash when you touch poison oak is their resin. They retain resin for years after they die. They contain as much resin in the winter as in the summer. If there is poison oak resin on your skin and you don't wash it off, by scratching your skin you can spread the resin to other parts of your body which could give you a painful rash all over. Wash every thing that has been in contact with the resin like clothes, towels, sheets, etc....to prevent such a rash.

My patient C. came to see me one day because her whole skin was itching. She was miserable. I examined her and discovered a big rash on her hands, arms, legs and belly. I asked her how it started. She said that it started "itching like crazy" 24 hours after she came back from a walk in the woods with her dog. She couldn't understand why. She had stayed on trails all the time, was fully dressed with heavy jeans and hiking shoes and hadn't come in contact with any plant. I asked her if her dog stayed on the trails too. She answered that her dog was off leash for 15 minutes and run wild in the woods during that time. It turned out that her dog ran in poison oak and had poison oak resin on his hair. When she petted him, she got this resin on her hands then touched her legs, arms and stomach with her hands which spread out the resin to a large part of her body. She only took a shower 6 hours later but didn't wash her dog. The following day, while petting her dog, she got in contact with more resin. That's when her rash got worse and her whole body started itching. I had her wash her dog and also wash every single thing her dog had been in contact with. I had to give her steroids to ease her pain but it took 2 weeks before she got completely back to normal. The moral of the story is: wash off any poison oak resin right away to prevent this kind of reaction.

Myth # 4:

After eating wild mushrooms picked up in the woods, the sooner you get nausea, vomiting and diarrhea the more serious the intoxication is. This is false. If you get vomiting and diarrhea within the first 2 hours, chances are that the intoxication won't be too serious. If vomiting and diarrhea start after 8 or even 10 to 16 hours after the intoxication, go to the emergency room right away. Wild mushrooms can be poisonous and cause liver failure and death. Do not eat wild mushrooms picked up in the woods.

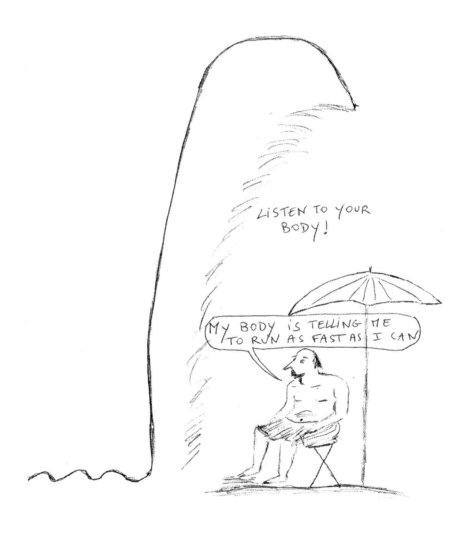

Chapter 23
Tools for prevention and early detection

*"He who has health has hope; and he who has hope
has everything."*

Arabic proverb

YOU are your own best primary care physician! As such, you need to constantly monitor all aspects of your body and observe any change that would warrant attention:

<u>Vision</u>

I recommend that on a regular basis, everyday when waking up, you make sure that your vision hasn't changed. Close your right eye and make sure you see far away and close up with your left eye. Make sure that when you look straight with the left eye, you see perfectly the whole field around you. Do the same thing with the other eye. Make sure the colors are not distorted. If at any time you see like a curtain coming down on your vision field or you have blurred vision in one eye becoming progressively worse, contact an eye specialist immediately. It could be a detached retina which is a surgical emergency. All persons over age 40 years should have intraocular pressure measurement and optic disc examination every 2-5 years. In diabetics and individuals with a family history of glaucoma, annual examination is indicated. Wear eye protection like glasses or goggles any time you do construction work, shoot guns or any time projectiles are at risk of being violently thrown in the air.

Hearing

Check how far from each ear you can hear 2 fingers rubbing against each other or a clock ticking. That distance should change very little over the years and should be symmetrical. If not symmetrical or if there is a decrease in hearing, consult your physician.

Make sure you wear ear protections around loud noises such as noisy machinery or shooting. Do not have loud music blasting in your ear, it could damage your hearing.

Skin

Examine your skin once a month to make sure there is no black or red lesion growing. A red lesion on the face, neck or chest could be a basal cell carcinoma which is a type of skin cancer that doesn't metastasize much. A change in a mole or a black lesion anywhere on your skin could be a melanoma which is a very dangerous type of skin cancer which could be deadly due to its metastasis. A black growing lesion which is larger than 5 mms diameter, has an irregular border and shape and different tones of black, brown, purple, red and white colors needs to be shown to a dermatologist as soon as possible. It could be a melanoma and needs to be taken out urgently. Don't forget to look in between your toes, on your nails, on your palms, soles and on your back.

Wear a hat, long sleeves shirt and long pants when in the sun between 10:00 am and 3:00 pm. Use sunscreen cream with an SPF of minimum 15. Use creams that contain physical blockers like Zinc Oxide and Titanium Dioxide or chemical blockers like Mexoryl that protects against UVAs and UVBs.

If you hurt yourself, apply pressure for 3 minutes right away.

If you have an open wound, disinfect it 2 or 3 times a day the first couple of days with hydrogen peroxide or povidone iodine.

Teeth

Floss and brush your teeth after each meal. Have your teeth cleaned and checked by a dentist twice a year. A new cavity needs to be treated by your dentist as soon as possible in order to prevent the loss of the tooth. If one tooth hurts when you eat something very cold like ice cream or something very hot like tea or coffee, it is indicative of a potentially serious problem that warrants an immediate appointment with your dentist.

Heart rate and blood pressure

Measurements by a physician in the office may not be the most accurate way to assess your blood pressure. Ambulatory monitoring and home self-measurements may be better. Getting a home blood pressure monitor is a wise investment. Use it in the morning when getting up and before dinner after 10 minutes of rest. It will tell you your systolic and diastolic blood pressure as well as your heart rate. Your blood pressure will show 2 numbers. The highest is called systolic and the lowest diastolic. Your blood pressure should be less than 120 mm Hg systolic and less than 80 mm Hg diastolic. If your systolic blood pressure is between 120 and 139 mm Hg or your diastolic blood pressure is between 80 and 89 mm Hg most of the days, you have pre-hypertension. If your systolic blood pressure is 140 mm Hg or over, you have hypertension. If your diastolic blood pressure is 90 mm Hg or over, you have hypertension also. If your are diabetic, have renal disease or cardiovascular disease, your blood pressure should be less than 130 mm Hg systolic and less than 85 mm Hg diastolic otherwise, you have hypertension. You don't need both numbers to be elevated; only one elevated number is enough to say you have high blood pressure. This means you have to start a low salt diet, reduce alcohol consumption, lose weight if you are overweight and exercise regularly. Have a diet high in fresh fruits and vegetable, low in fat, red meats and sugar-containing beverages.

Add a little piece of dark chocolate everyday without exceeding 7 oz in a week. If all this fails, you need a prescription medical treatment every day to decrease your blood pressure. Otherwise you could be at risk for stroke.

If you are a man over 40 or a woman over 50, you might benefit from taking one baby aspirin every day (81 mg). It will prevent your blood from getting too thick and make blood clots.

Monitor your urine color and stool color regularly.

The color of your urine and stools is a great indicator of a potentially serious problem. Any indication of blood in urine or stools warrants an immediate visit to your doctor.

After age 50, get a colonoscopy to make sure you don't have any colon polyp. Then get a colonoscopy every 10 years until age 75 if no polyp is found after the first colonoscopy. Get a colonoscopy every 3 years if a polyp is found. Colonoscopies allow polyps to be removed and questionable lesions to be biopsied. It allows early detection of colon cancer. Early detection allows early treatment which most often permits a complete resection and cure. Virtual colonoscopies are less aggressive for the body but they do not allow any biopsy.

If anybody in your immediate family had colon cancer before age 60, start having colonoscopy yourself 10 years before that age.

Make sure your vaccinations are up to date. Since recommended vaccinations are updated regularly, check with your doctor which ones you need. You can also check online at www.cdc.gov/vaccines.

Mainly, you should get protected against Diphteria, Tetanus (every 10 years), Pertussis, Haemophilus Influenzae type B, Varicella, Measles, Mumps, Rubella, Hepatitis A and B.

A new vaccination is the HPV (Human Papillomavirus) immunization which should be given to all preadolescent girls before the onset of sexual activity and to other female patients up to 26 years of age who wish to reduce their risk of HPV infection (which cause most cases of cervical cancer and genital warts). HPV disease is the most common sexually transmitted disease in the United States.

Also get a flu shot every year.

After age 60, in addition, get a Zoster (shingles) vaccine and after age 65, a Pneumococcal vaccine.

If you are planning to travel to developing countries, check online at www.cdc.gov/travel for advice on immunizations and travel-related health problems.

<u>Sex</u>

There are a lot of sexually transmitted diseases out there. If you are having a new sex partner, use condoms plus lubricants. Your partner can look really healthy and yet be HIV positive, hepatitis C positive, have gonorrhea or syphilis. Just one sexual encounter can contaminate you. Your partner can have genital herpes and contaminate you even if the last outbreak was months ago. Remember that one moment of sexual pleasure with the wrong person could create a lifetime of painful disease and premature death. It could also result in an unwanted pregnancy. Get to know your partner really well and don't be afraid to ask for an HIV, syphilis and hepatitis C test before you have sex.

<u>For women,</u> examine your breasts yourself once a month, making sure there is no lump. If you feel a new lump, consult your physician immediately. Between 20 and 40 years old, get a clinical breast examination by a physician every 3 years. After 40 years old, get a yearly physical examination and some physicians say you need to start getting a mammogram every couple of years. After 50 years old, get a mammogram every year or couple of years. Mammograms allow detection of tiny calcifications and small tumors. A mammogram might detect breast cancer before it can be felt through palpation.

For breast cancer, early detection and early treatment are keys for a complete cure.

Have regular pap (Papanicolaou test) smears and HPV (Human Papillomavirus) tests for early detection of cervix of the uterus cancer. Have a pap smear every year beginning within 3 years after your first vaginal intercourse and no later than age 21. After age 30, women with three normal tests and a negative HPV test may be screened every 2-3 years. After age 70, you may choose to stop screening if you have had three normal and no abnormal pap smear within the last 10 years.

For men, after 50 years old, have your doctor examine your prostate through a digital rectal exam and do a PSA (prostate-specific antigen) blood test once a year to detect prostate cancer early.

Feet and hands

Wear open shoes at home. Some people only wear tennis shoes. They wear tennis shoes at work, at home and in the evening when they go out. They only take their closed tennis shoes off a few hours at night. This is a perfect recipe for a great fungus farm. I bet their fungus pets on their feet are very happy. In order not to grow any fungus, wear open shoes at home. When you are out, alternate shoes; sometimes wear leather shoes, sometimes tennis shoes. Don't wear every day the same shoes. If you tend to sweat a lot, use over-the-counter antifungal powder in your closed shoes at least once a week. It will prevent your unwanted fungus pets to feel at home in your shoes.

When working in your yard, use heavy gloves to protect your fingers and wear closed shoes to protect your feet. If you walk in the countryside and through woods, wear long pants and high ankle shoes to protect your skin from poison oak. Know what poison oak looks like. If your skin was in contact with poison oak, the first thing to do it to wash the plant resin off with soap and water. People that are allergic to poison oak have around two hours to do so before their skin starts reacting. Also wash the clothes that have been in contact with the resin. Poison oak is widely present in the whole United States and about 50% of people are allergic to its resin.

When working at your computer:

Make sure that your back is straight at all times and that your wrists are not bent. Get up every hour to stretch. Get up every couple of hours to do at least 10 minutes of physical exercise. The worse possible position for your back is sitting down for long hours without moving. It is a very common cause of backache. As for your wrists, if they are bent for long hours, you could get carpel tunnel syndrome.

First aid kit

Have a first aid kit at home. This should include:

Povidone iodine to disinfect scrapes and wounds (very potent but tends to stain).

Hydrogen Peroxide to disinfect scrapes and wounds (less potent but doesn't stain)

Arnica cream or gel to use on hematomas

Triple antibiotic cream for wounds or burns.

1% hydrocortisone cream for itchy bug bites.

Sterile eye saline which can be used to rinse your eyes and also to wash any wound.

Band-aids of different sizes.

Blood pressure monitor.

Thermometer to check your fever.

Ace wrapping for ankle or knee sprain.

Magnifying glass, a bottle of alcohol and a sterile needle to take splinters out of your body.

Conclusion

"There is nothing noble about being superior to some other person. The true nobility is being superior to your previous self."

Hindustani proverb

Medicine is not only a science, it is an art. Healthy living is also an art.

As we have shown in this book, it takes time to find the right balance for you. It takes energy to find the right foods, beverages, sleep pattern, physical exercise, friends, partner and passion in life. It takes knowledge, wisdom and common sense to detect and treat early any abnormal symptom. Know that things can and will change and that you need to reevaluate the right balance for you every few years. As you go through different phases of your life from childhood to adolescence, from early adulthood to midlife to senior life, your body will metabolize foods differently. Chances are, as you get older towards midlife and especially as you become a senior citizen, you will need to eat less to avoid gaining weight. Your mind will become more mature and your needs and goals in life will change. You need to rebalance your life periodically. You need to listen to your body regularly.

Once you have found how to be healthy and balanced, once you understand what you body is trying to tell you when it screams, it will be a gold mine for the rest of your life. You will feel so much better. Instead of having to take a lot of medications to treat diseases and having to spend a lot of money on blood tests, radiology tests and doctors office visits, you will be able to prevent diseases. This primary prevention will allow you and your insurance to save a lot of money. It will enable you to help others. Above all, it will allow you to teach these extremely precious skills to your children. Without these skills, their life could be in danger. Being a good parent is an art. One out of 3 children born this year will be diabetic. This is an enormous number! A lot of parents feed their children the wrong foods! We have seen 4 year old children weighing more than 150 lbs without having any medical disorder. They were just not exercising at all and were eating high calorie processed foods all the time. This was destroying their lives and their health.

Do not destroy your perfect body! Do not ruin your children's life! Teach them at an early age the A, B, C's of a healthy life. Teach them how to listen to their body. They will be eternally grateful to you

As for you, this will allow you to have a wonderful, balanced, long and exciting life!

Bibliography

Natural Baby and childcare by Lauren Feder, MD (healthy living books 2006)

The second brain by Michael D. Gershon, MD (HarperCollins 1998)

Homeopathic Therapeutics: Possibilities in Acute Pathology by Jacques Jouanny, MD, Jean-Bernard Crapanne, MD, Henry Dancer, MD, Jean-Louis Masson, MD (Editions Boiron 1996)

Homeopathic Therapeutics: Possibilities in Chronic Pathology by Jacques Jouanny, MD, Jean-Bernard Crapanne, MD, Henry Dancer, MD, Jean-Louis Masson, MD (Editions Boiron 1994)

Pharmacology and Homeopathic Materia Medica by Denis Demarque, MD, Jacques Jouanny, MD, Bernard Poitevin, MD, Yves Saint-Jean MD (Editions Boiron, 1997)

Tantra, the art of conscious loving by Charles and Caroline Muir (Mercury House 1989).

Lancet, 2006; 368(9529):83-86 Are *statins analogues of vitamin D?* by Grimes DS

Front Biosci, 2005; 10:2723-2749 *Vitamin D and cancer: an update of in vitro and in vivo data* by Ordonez-Moran P, Larriba MJ, Pendas-Franco N, et al.

J. Steroid Biochemistry Molecular Biology 2006: 102 (1-5): 156-162 *Vitamin D and cancer* by Bouillon R, Eelen G, Verlinden L, Mathieu C, Carmeliet G, Verstuyf A

Diabetes Care, 2006: 29(3): 650-656 *Vitamin D and calcium intake in relation to type 2 diabetes in women* by Pittas AG, Dawson-Hughes B, Li T, et al.